Hillcrest Medical Center

Beginning Medical Transcription Course

Fifth Edition

Mary Ann Novak, Ph.D.
Associate Professor
Information Management Systems
College of Applied Sciences and Arts
Southern Illinois University
Carbondale, Illinois

Patricia A. Ireland, CMT
Medical Transcriptionist, Freelance Author, Medical/Technical Editor
San Antonio, Texas

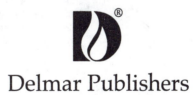

Delmar Publishers

an International Thomson Publishing company I(T)P®

Albany • Bonn • Boston • Cincinnati • Detroit • London • Madrid
Melbourne • Mexico City • New York • Pacific Grove • Paris • San Francisco
Singapore • Tokyo • Toronto • Washington

NOTICE TO THE READER

Cover Design: Brucie Rosch

Delmar Staff:
Publisher: Susan Simpfenderfer
Acquisitions Editor: Marlene McHugh Pratt
Developmental Editor: Jill Rembetski
Project Editor: William Trudell
Art and Design Coordinator: Rich Killar
Production Coordinator: Rich Killar
Marketing Manager: Darryl L. Caron
Editorial Assistant: Maria Perretta

COPYRIGHT © 1999
By Delmar Publishers Inc.
a division of International Thomson Publishing Inc.

The ITP logo is a trademark under license.

Printed in the United States of America

For more information, contact:

Delmar Publishers
3 Columbia Circle, Box 15015
Albany, New York 12212-5015

International Thomson Publishing Europe
Berkshire House 168-173
High Holborn
London, WC1V 7AA
England

Thomas Nelson Australia
102 Dodds Street
South Melbourne, 3205
Victoria, Australia

Nelson Canada
1120 Birchmount Road
Scarborough, Ontario
Canada, M1K 5G4

International Thomson Editores
Campos Eliseos 385, Piso 7
Col Polanco
11560 Mexico D F Mexico

International Thomson Publishing GmbH
Konigswinterer Strasse 418
53227 Bonn
Germany

International Thomson Publishing Asia
221 Henderson Road
#05-10 Henderson Building
Singapore 0315

International Thomson Publishing—Japan
Hirakawacho Kyowa Building, 3F
2-2-1 Hirakawacho
Chiyoda-ku, Tokyo 102
Japan

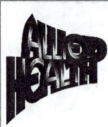

JOIN US ON THE WEB: www.DelmarAlliedHealth.com

Your Information Resource!
• What's New from Delmar • Health Science News Headlines
• Web Links to Many Related Sites
• Instructor Forum/Teaching Tips • Give Us Your Feedback
• Online Companions™
• Complete Allied Health Catalog • Software/Media Demos
• And much more!

A service of I**T**P®

1 2 3 4 5 6 7 8 9 10 XXX 04 03 02 01 00 99 98 98

Novak, Mary Ann, 1944-
    Hillcrest medical Center : beginning medical transcription course
/ Mary Ann Novak, Patricia A. Ireland — 5th ed.
        p.   cm.
    Includes bibliographical references and index.
    ISBN 0–7668–0322–8
    1. Medical transcription.   I. Ireland, Patricia A. 1940-
II. Hillcrest Medical Center (Miami, Fla.) III. Title.
    [DNLM: 1. Medical records. 2. Medical records problems.
3. Nomenclature. 4. Nomenclature problems. WX 173 N936h 1999]
R728.8.N68   1999
651.5' 02461--dc21
DNLM/DLC
for Library of Congress

651.961
N935

98-16973
CIP

Contents

Preface

Hillcrest Medical Center: Beginning Medical Transcription Course is a text-workbook created to introduce students to the interesting and challenging world of medical transcription. The contents of the text-workbook are designed to familiarize students with eight basic medical reports concerning Hillcrest Medical Center inpatients and two basic medical reports concerning Quali-Care Clinic outpatients, related medical terminology, an appropriate format for transcribing the reports, and specialized rules of grammar and punctuation peculiar to dictated medical reports. Users will apply these principles as they transcribe the medical reports that comprise the 10 case studies relating to inpatients and the 20 medical reports relating to outpatients.

Students of the *Hillcrest Medical Center* textbook and tapes learn through a well-rounded course of beginning medical dictation and transcription. After the completion of this textbook, students may progress to the advanced dictation available through *Forrest General Medical Center: Advanced Medical Terminology and Transcription Course*, 2nd edition textbook and tapes. This advanced text goes into more detailed specialty and subspecialty dictation. The *Forrest General* text is strongly recommended to round out the medical transcription students' experience and to prepare them for employment.

PREREQUISITES

Students should be proficient in keyboarding and have a working knowledge of transcription equipment before beginning this course. Even though a section of the text-workbook relates to understanding medical terminology, it is strongly suggested that students complete a course in medical terminology before beginning *Hillcrest Medical Center.*

COURSE DESCRIPTION

This is a beginning medical transcription course designed to provide students with a working knowledge of the transcription of medical reports. Medical reports will be transcribed from 10 individual case studies, each of which concerns an inpatient with a specific medical problem. There are between three and eight reports within each case study. The case studies have been taken from hospital medical records. Students will be involved in the care of the patient from the date of admission to Hillcrest Medical Center through the date of discharge. The eight medical reports included are history and physical examinations, radiology reports, operative reports, pathology reports, requests for consultation, death summaries, discharge summaries, and autopsy reports. Following are the case numbers and related specialty areas.

Case 1: Reproductive System
Case 2: Musculoskeletal System
Case 3: Cardiovascular System
Case 4: Integumentary System
Case 5: Urinary System
Case 6: Nervous System
Case 7: Digestive System
Case 8: Endocrine System
Case 9: Lymphatic System
Case 10: Respiratory System

In addition, 20 outpatient medical reports will be transcribed, each of which concerns a patient with a specific medical problem and who was treated by a physician at Quali-Care Clinic. The outpatient reports, generally referred to as the HPIP (history, physical, impression, plan) and the SOAP (subjective, objective, assessment, plan) formats, have been taken from actual patient medical records. Following are the report numbers and related specialty areas:

Report 1: Radiology
Report 2: Orthopedics
Report 3: Neurology
Report 4: Gastroenterology
Report 5: Dermatology
Report 6: Family Practice
Report 7: Genitourinary
Report 8: Rheumatology
Report 9: Dermatology
Report 10: Radiology
Report 11: Family Practice
Report 12: Gastroenterology
Report 13: Cardiology
Report 14: Family Practice
Report 15: Psychiatry

Report 16: Dermatology
Report 17: Genitourinary
Report 18: Pulmonology
Report 19: Psychiatry
Report 20: Obstetrics

COURSE DESIGN

These materials are designed to be used in a traditional classroom setting scheduled to meet at designated times each week. Laboratory time is scheduled either individually or in groups, and students report during their assigned lab time. It is up to each instructor to decide whether or not to be present in the lab. The estimated time to complete the case studies is 32 class hours (2 days per week for 16 weeks), plus additional laboratory time to transcribe the medical reports (approximately 3-6 hours per case study). Transcription time will vary depending on the length of the case study, the student's keyboarding skills, and the student's command of the English language. Additional lab hours should be assigned to transcribe the 20 outpatient medical reports.

These materials would also be effective in a hospital in-service education department. New employees or those being cross-trained or retrained could complete all of the case studies plus the outpatient reports. Those who are interested in a particular medical specialty could transcribe the reports relative to that specialty area. However, transcription laboratory time should be provided, allowing the employees to work at their own pace.

OBJECTIVES

Upon successful completion of this course, students should be able to do the following:

1. Describe the importance of the confidential nature of medical reports.

2. Describe the content and purpose of the eight inpatient medical reports used at Hillcrest Medical Center.

3. Describe the content and purpose of the 20 outpatient medical reports used at Quali-Care Clinic.

4. Transcribe medical reports using correct report format.

5. Transcribe medical reports using correct capitalization, number, punctuation, abbreviation, symbol, and metric measurement rules.

6. Spell correctly both the English and medical terms and abbreviations presented, either by memory or by using a dictionary/reference book.

7. Define the medical terms and abbreviations presented, either by memory or by using a dictionary/reference book.

8. Define the prefixes, combining forms, and suffixes presented.

9. Identify and define the knowledge, skills, abilities, and responsibilities required of a medical transcriptionist.

10. Recognize the advantages of having current reference material and be able to use it effectively.

11. Use standard proofreader's marks to edit medical reports without changing the meaning or the dictator's style.

These objectives can be achieved by reading the material presented in the text-workbook, by transcribing the medical reports, and by completing the proofreading exercises.

STUDENT TEXT-WORKBOOK

Introduction

The introduction consists of both a welcome letter addressed to students and the confidentiality policy for Hillcrest Medical Center. The purpose of the letter is to inform students about their position as a medical transcriptionist at Hillcrest and to emphasize the importance of the medical transcriptionist's role in healthcare. The letter also describes Hillcrest as a specific medical facility. The "Confidentiality Policy" explains how important it is for employees at Hillcrest to understand and maintain confidentiality of patient records.

Information on the American Association for Medical Transcription (AAMT), a national association representing the medical transcription profession, is also presented in this section. The "AAMT Model Job Description" for medical transcriptionists includes information about the knowledge, skills, and abilities required of medical transcriptionists, as well as the job responsibilities and performance standards of medical transcriptionists.

The "AAMT Code of Ethics" is presented with information about the AAMT national certification examination.

Understanding Medical Records

The content and purpose of the eight model inpatient medical report forms used at Hillcrest Medical Center are discussed in this section.

Transcription Rules for Hillcrest

Rules pertaining to capitalization, numbers, punctuation, abbreviations, and symbols used to create medical reports at both Hillcrest Medical Center and Quali-Care Clinic are discussed.

Case Studies

Students will be required to complete 10 case studies. Each case study consists of:

1. A scenario including the inpatient's name and address, a summary of the inpatient's medical problem, the various specialists involved in the inpatient's care, and a list of specific reports involved.

2. A glossary of medical terms used in each case study that includes definitions and phonetic pronunciations.

3. Pertinent illustrations.

Outpatient Reports

Students will also be required to complete 20 outpatient reports. Information about each outpatient includes:

1. The patient's name with a brief description of the patient's illness.

2. A glossary of medical terms used in each outpatient report that includes definitions and pronunciations.

Audiocassettes

The reports related to each inpatient case are recorded on cassette to be transcribed by the students. The terms listed in each glossary are dictated, followed by the medical report dictation. Cases 1-5 contain timed dictation at 80 and 90 words per minute; case 6-10 contain office-style dictation. Different regional accents and background noises that duplicate real-life situations are used in the recorded dictation. The 10 transcription tests are

dictated using the same speed and style as their corresponding case tapes.

The reports related to each outpatient are also recorded on cassette to be transcribed by the students. The terms listed in each glossary are dictated, followed by the medical report dictation. Reports 1–10 contain timed dictation at 80 and 90 words per minute; reports 11–20 contain office-style dictation. Different regional accents and background noises that duplicate real-life situations are used in the recorded dictation. The five transcription tests are dictated using the same speed and style as the 20 outpatient medical reports; i.e., transcription test 1 is dictated at 80 words per minute, transcription test 2 is dictated at 90 words per minute, and transcription tests 3, 4, and 5 contain office-style dictation.

Skill-Building Exercises

Additional exercises are included in the Appendix to strengthen students' skills in medical transcription. These include proofreading exercises and crossword puzzles.

Appendix

The following helpful information is also included in the Appendix:

1. Proofreader's marks

2. Challenging medical words, phrases, and prefixes

3. Lund Browder burn chart

4. Reference material, publishers, and internet addresses

5. Healthcare Controlled Vocabulary

Index

The words, phrases, and abbreviations listed in each glossary are presented in alphabetic order in the index, along with the case number or report number in which they were introduced. The prefixes, combining forms, and suffixes are also included; the page numbers identify their first location in the text-workbook.

INSTRUCTOR'S MANUAL

A comprehensive Instructor's Manual is available that discusses the design of the course, suggestions for teaching the course, evaluation procedures, and production standards. Transcripts for the 10 inpatient case studies and the 20 outpatient medical reports are provided in the manual, as well as a test bank that includes:

1. Ten written quizzes plus the answer keys, which correlate with the 10 inpatient case studies.

2. The answer keys to 10 transcription tests relating to inpatient case studies, which are recorded on cassettes.

3. The answer keys to five transcription tests relating to outpatients, which are recorded on cassettes.

4. Answer keys to the proofreading exercises, word find exercises (contained on student disk), and crossword puzzles.

A "Certificate of Completion," which is to be given to the student on successful completion of *Hillcrest Medical Center*, is also included in the manual.

Acknowledgments

This text-workbook is the result of the cooperation and input of many individuals. The authors would like to express their appreciation for authentic medical reports submitted for adaptation and inclusion in this text-workbook. Additionally, the authors want to thank the reviewers for their contributions and suggestions. Their feedback enabled us to develop a text-workbook to better serve your needs.

Linda Andrews
Director
The Andrews School
Oklahoma City, OK

Shirley S. Gordon
Instructor
Ascension College
Gonzales, LA

Brenda Potter
Medical Secretary Instructor
Moorhead Northwest Technical Institute
Fargo, ND

Esther Storvold
Selkirk College
Trail, BC

Barbara Thomas
Salisbury Business College
Salisbury, NC

Mary Walker
Southwestern Technical College
Jackson, MN

ABOUT THE AUTHORS

Patricia A. Ireland, CMT, has been a medical transcriptionist since 1968. She has 10 years' experience as a part-time instructor of medical transcription and medical terminology at the community college level. She works as a medical transcriptionist and a freelance medical/technical editor in San Antonio, Texas.

Mary Ann Novak, Ph.D., has been teaching office professionals for 18 years and is an Associate Professor in the Department of Information Management Systems, College of Applied Sciences and Arts, Southern Illinois University, Carbondale, Illinois.

Introduction

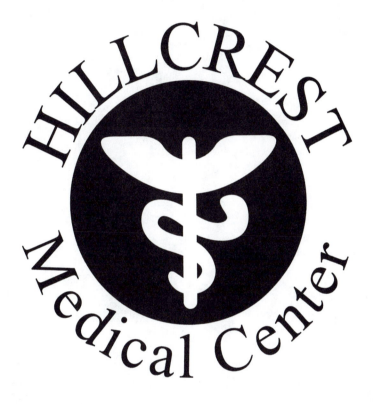

Welcome to Hillcrest Medical Center

You are now employed as a medical transcriptionist (MT) in the medical records department at Hillcrest Medical Center, transcribing reports for patients admitted to Hillcrest Medical Center and transcribing outpatients reports for patients treated at Quali-Care Clinic. MTs are a vital part of the healthcare team because physicians and allied health professionals rely on medical records, legal documents subject to subpoena, to maintain and document proper patient care. Because of the confidential nature of these medical records, you will be asked to read the "Confidentiality Policy" on page 000 and sign the "Confidentiality Statement" before beginning your duties at Hillcrest.

During your employment at Hillcrest, you will be transcribing medical reports from 10 individual case studies, each relating to an inpatient with a specific medical problem. The case studies have been taken from actual hospital medical records, and you will be involved in the care of each patient from the date of admission to Hillcrest through the date of discharge. The eight medical reports that you will be transcribing include history and physical examinations, radiology reports, operative reports, pathology reports, requests for consultation, discharge summaries, death summaries, and autopsy reports.

Presented on the first page of each case study is a brief scenario including the patient's name and address, a summary of the patient's medical problem, the various specialists involved in the patient's care, and a list of the specific reports involved. In addition, a glossary of medical terms is provided for each case study. Each glossary includes phonetic pronunciations with definitions for the medical terms, phrases, and abbreviations used in each case study.

The MTs who are employed by Hillcrest will also transcribe dictated tapes for the healthcare providers who maintain offices at Quali-Care Clinic. This service is provided as a courtesy to the staff of Quali-Care Clinic, a freestanding medical office facility on the grounds of Hillcrest Medical Center. With the changes in insurance, the advent of health management organizations, preferred provider organizations, and managed care, the Hillcrest Medical Center Board of Directors voted to have Quali-Care Clinic built to treat a burgeoning number of outpatients—those who have no need for either inpatient care or emergency room care.

The performance evaluations in this text-workbook will consist of transcription tests and written quizzes. Therefore, it is important to learn the information presented in each case study and medical report, including appropriate report format and transcription rules observed by the Hillcrest medical records department. Before transcribing the medical reports, become familiar with the spellings, pronunciations, and definitions of the terms and abbreviations presented in the glossaries. Words are "tools of the trade" for MTs.

Hillcrest Medical Center is a 400-bed general community hospital located in Miami, Florida. All patient services, the emergency room, and the surgery suite are found on the first and second floors. On the third floor, there are beds for 60 inpatients—20 in the pediatric unit, 20 in the coronary care unit (CCU), and 20 in the intensive care unit (ICU). Pediatric patients are usually those 14 years of age or younger. CCU is for patients—medical or surgical—who are seriously ill with heart disease; an ICU patient would be someone who is either gravely ill or has had surgery on a weekend or a holiday. Otherwise, the postoperative patients are sent to the fourth floor where there are 100 beds for surgical patients. The fifth floor has 100 beds used for medical patients, and the sixth floor has 100 beds used for geriatric patients or for those who need long-term care.

From time to time Hillcrest accepts patients transferred from Forrest General Hospital, the county hospital and teaching facility for the local medical school. Hillcrest sometimes sends patients to Forrest General for specific evaluations, for consultations, or for certain sophisticated procedures not available at Hillcrest.

We look forward to a pleasant working relationship, and we hope your employment as an MT at Hillcrest Medical Center proves to be a rewarding experience.

Sincerely,

Allison Poole

Allison Poole, CMT, RRA
Director, Medical Records Department

CONFIDENTIALITY POLICY

The primary purpose of the medical record is to document the course of a patient's illness and treatment during all periods of the patient's care. The medical record is extremely important as a permanent account of the patient care provided. It serves as a means of communication between physicians and other healthcare professionals. As such, it is also a tool for planning and evaluating patient care.

For the medical record to be a useful instrument in patient care, it must contain accurate, detailed, personal information relating to each patient's medical, surgical, psychiatric, social, and family history.

Patients have the **right** to expect their medical records to be treated as **confidential**, and Hillcrest Medical Center personnel have an **obligation** to safeguard patients' medical records against unauthorized disclosure.

As an employee of Hillcrest Medical Center, you have a responsibility to ensure that each patient's right to privacy is safeguarded. You will have direct access to information contained in medical records. Information learned during the course of your work **must** be held in strictest confidence.

To ensure the confidentiality of patient information, employees of Hillcrest Medical Center must sign a statement acknowledging this Confidentiality Policy. Violations of this policy will result in immediate disciplinary action.

Confidentiality Statement

I,_____, an employee of Hillcrest Medical Center, have read and reviewed the Confidentiality Policy with my supervisor. I understand the importance of each employee complying with this policy. I further understand that if I intentionally violate this policy by any unauthorized release of a patient's medical information, this violation could constitute grounds for my immediate dismissal.

_____   _____
Date   Signature of Employee

_____   _____
Date   Witness

LEGAL ISSUES

In creating these medical reports, which are legal documents, what do you do if dictation is unintelligible or a section of tape is blank? Students and experienced MTs both encounter dictation that cannot be understood, and a directive should be in place in each MT's office or workplace in this event. Some suggestions follow:

1. If you encounter a word or phrase that cannot be understood, look it up in your reference material. This would include dictionaries, word books, drug books, and other lists of medical words/phrases. (See Reference Material, page 41.)

2. If you are unsuccessful in locating the word or phrase in the reference material, have your supervisor or a coworker listen to the difficult section of dictation. One of them may be able to interpret the word or phrase.

3. If these two options are unsuccessful, the report should be flagged for the originator's attention. An underlined blank (____) should *always* be left when dictation is left out of a report. This lets anyone who comes in contact with the report know that there is a question about the dictation—words to be filled in—and the originator of the report is the one to fill in the word(s).

A telephone call to the doctor's office could possibly yield results; however, this is not always feasible. As you work in the field of medical transcription, you will learn different "tricks of the trade" that can be used. As beginners, however, you must follow your supervisor's lead. The ideal report, of course, has no blanks; however, this situation is often out of the MT's control. Even so, you should not make up words to avoid leaving a blank. Even experienced MTs leave blanks from time to time.

The physician who originates the report and whose signature is on it is the party legally responsible for the contents thereof. This means that each report should be carefully read by the originator, corrected in the computer, reprinted, then signed as corrected. Unfortunately, this is another situation that is not within the MT's control. The originator may make handwritten corrections on the report that never get back to the transcriptionist and, therefore, never get entered into the computer. Also, many reports are signed without being read at all. So, even though the physician who signs it is legally responsible, more and more MTs are buying liability insurance to cover themselves in case of a lawsuit. (The cost for this insurance would be a valid business tax deduction.)

OBJECTIVES

At Hillcrest Medical Center students learn how to transcribe medical reports. During the transcription process, students will increase their medical vocabulary, use an appropriate format for transcribing the reports, and apply specialized rules of grammar and punctuation peculiar to dictated medical reports. Upon successful completion of this course, students should be able to do the following:

1. Describe the importance of the confidential nature of medical records.

2. Describe the content and purpose of the eight medical inpatient reports used at Hillcrest Medical Center.

3. Describe the content and purpose of the two outpatient medical reports used at Quali-Care Clinic.

4. Transcribe medical reports using correct report format.

5. Transcribe medical reports using correct capitalization, number, punctuation, abbreviation, symbol, and metric measurement rules.

6. Spell correctly both the English and medical terms and abbreviations presented, either by memory or by using a dictionary/reference book.

7. Define the medical terms and abbreviations presented, either by memory or by using a dictionary/reference book.

8. Define the prefixes, combining forms, and suffixes presented.

9. Identify and define the knowledge, skills, abilities, and responsibilities required of an MT.

10. Recognize the advantages of having current reference material and be able to use it effectively.

11. Use standard proofreader's marks to edit medical reports without changing the meaning or the originator's style.

These objectives can be achieved by reading the material presented in the text-workbook, by transcribing the medical reports, and by completing the proofreading exercises.

LENGTH OF COURSE

Students will be required to complete the ten inpatient case studies listed below. The time estimated to complete the case studies is 32 class hours (2 days per week for 16 weeks), plus additional laboratory time to transcribe the medical reports (approximately 3-6 hours per case study). Transcription time will vary depending on the length of the case study, the student's keyboarding skills, and the student's command of English language usage and punctuation.

Case 1: Reproductive System
Case 2: Musculoskeletal System
Case 3: Cardiovascular System
Case 4: Integumentary System
Case 5: Urinary System
Case 6: Nervous System
Case 7: Digestive System
Case 8: Endocrine System
Case 9: Lymphatic System
Case 10: Respiratory System

Additional laboratory time should be allotted to the students to transcribe 20 outpatient medical reports, each of which concerns a patient with a specific medical problem that was treated by a physician at Quali-Care Clinic. The outpatient reports, generally referred to as the HPIP (history, physical, impression, plan) and the SOAP (subjective, objective, assessment, plan) formats, have been taken from actual patient medical records. Following are the report numbers and related specialty areas:

Report 1: Radiology
Report 2: Orthopedics
Report 3: Neurology
Report 4: Gastroenterology
Report 5: Dermatology
Report 6: Family Practice
Report 7: Genitourinary
Report 8: Rheumatology
Report 9: Dermatology
Report 10: Radiology
Report 11: Family Practice

Report 12: Gastroenterology
Report 13: Cardiology
Report 14: Family Practice
Report 15: Psychiatry
Report 16: Dermatology
Report 17: Genitourinary
Report 18: Pulmonology
Report 19: Psychiatry
Report 20: Obstetrics

Certification

The word "certification" is used in different ways. A certificate of completion is offered after almost any course that one may take. This certifies that you have completed the required course work, and it may be beneficial to have for your résumé or your personnel file. It does not mean, however, that you are a certified medical transcriptionist (CMT).

Certification by your professional association, which for MTs is the American Association for Medical Transcription in Modesto, California, is much different. Status as a certified medical transcriptionist (CMT) is earned by passing both the written and the practical examinations offered by the Medical Transcriptionist Certification Program (MTCP) through AAMT. Certification is retained by earning 30 continuing education credits every 3 years, which are reported to the MTCP on forms sent out for this purpose.

Certification by MTCP is not required to either be a member of AAMT or to work in the field of medical transcription. It is, however, a mark of quality and professionalism that indicates a dedication to continuing education.

TRANSCRIBING MEDICAL REPORTS

"In its basic unadulterated form, a medical record is an objective recording of the patient's clinical course progressing from evaluation and diagnosis to treatment and response. The medical record reflects the physician's thoughts and management of the clinical problem. If it is not recorded, it was not thought or done. The medical record is the foundation of good medical practice. After all of the skilled emergency management, complex and difficult diagnostic studies, and magnificent surgery, the clear, accurately recorded medical record is all that remains to confirm what was done or not done. This fundamental principle is learned by every student of medicine."[1]

Review the following information prior to transcribing the medical reports presented in this text-workbook.

1. Become familiar with both the content and format of the Hillcrest Medical Center inpatient model report forms. Also become familiar with both the content and format of the Quali-Care Clinic outpatient model report forms. The structure of outpatient and inpatient medical reports will vary among healthcare facilities.

2. Become familiar with the prefixes, combining forms, and suffixes that begin on page 57.

3. Learn the spelling and definition of the medical terms, phrases, and abbreviations presented in the glossary preceding each inpatient case study and each outpatient medical report. The glossaries in the case studies and medical reports are cumulative. Medical terms/abbreviations can have more than one meaning and more than one pronunciation; the definitions presented here pertain to the Hillcrest case studies and the Quali-Care medical reports.

4. The medical terms, phrases, and abbreviations appearing in the glossaries are dictated on the cassette tapes that accompany the text-workbook. Listen to the pronunciation of these terms prior to transcribing each case study. Take time to become familiar with the sound of each word.

5. The pronunciation of most medical terms is indicated by a phonetic respelling that appears in parentheses immediately following each term in the glossary. *Note:* Some words have more than one pronunciation, which is indicated.

6. Prior to transcribing, review the rules of capitalization, numbers, punctuation, abbreviations, and symbols on pages 41–47. These rules are not all inclusive,

---

[1]Used with permission from *CENTRAL FLORIDA PHYSICIAN*, the magazine of the Orange County Medical Society, Orlando, Florida 32804.

and it is recommended that you use one of the standard grammar reference books, a partial list of which appears in the Appendix on page 222.

7. Maintain at least one-inch side margins and one-inch top and bottom margins on each transcribed page.

8. If an inpatient medical report consists of more than one page, each succeeding page should have a heading at the left margin to include the name of the report. (See model reports for an example of a second-page heading.) If an outpatient medical report consists of more than one page, each succeeding page should have a heading that includes patient name, date seen, and page number. Second and third page headings may vary among healthcare facilities.

9. At the end of each report, key a signature line for the physician who dictated the report. Transcriptionist sign-off information consists of the reference initials of both the originator and transcriptionist, the date the report was dictated (D), and the date transcribed (T). This is keyed at the left margin two spaces below the signature line. (See model reports for an example of a signature line and transcriptionist sign-off information.)

10. In the case of pathology reports, the gross description is usually done on the day of scheduled surgery. The microscopic description and diagnosis are done after the tissue removed at surgery has been properly processed (at least 24 hours later). Therefore, the reference initials and dates dictated and transcribed are recorded after the gross description and again after the microscopic description and diagnosis. The physician and MT for the two descriptions may be the same or they may be altogether different. Whether the same or different physicians dictate the gross description and the microscopic description, two sets of reference initials and dates are required with one signature line at the end of the report. (See pathology model report.)

EVALUATIONS

Upon completion of each inpatient case study, you are required to take a written quiz that consists of the terms and their definitions as presented in each glossary. Each quiz is worth 20 points.

Ten transcription tests that relate to inpatients at Hillcrest and five transcription tests that relate to outpatients at Quali-Care Clinic are included on cassettes. Your instructor will decide when to administer the transcription tests; however, it is advisable for students to have transcribed and received feedback on at least the first two inpatient case studies and the first five outpatient reports before being assigned a transcription test.

SKILL-BUILDING EXERCISES

Several types of skill-building exercises have been provided to increase your skills in medical transcription. These exercises are described below.

Word Find Exercises/Crossword Puzzles

In keeping with the idea of being "word people," or those who find pleasure in working with and playing with words, Hillcrest offers word games. More than just games, they reinforce knowledge of terms presented in the text glossaries in a pleasant, stimulating way.

These word find exercises (found on the student disk) and crossword puzzles are offered as an alternative to be used during class time as a group activity. They are not intended to be used as testing material or as homework assignments but are offered as an activity to be completed from memory.

They also may be used as an exercise for beginning MT students to practice the use of their medical and pharmaceutical reference material.

Proofreading Exercises

"Detail oriented" is a phrase that describes an MT. "Focal" and "word person" are others. In creating and editing medical records, students should strive to become detail-oriented, focal workers.

There are several key decisions made by the MT at work. They include choosing the correct medical word by meaning and context, the correct spelling for both medical terms and English words, the correct format according to institution or client, punctuation, grammar, spacing, styling of numbers and symbols, PLUS editing, i.e., making additions and deletions without changing either the meaning or the originator's style.

To help beginning MT students become focal, detail-oriented professionals, Hillcrest offers a set of proofreading exercises. Errors incorporated into these exercises include examples of all the key decisions to be made by an MT. The standard proofreader's marks are printed on page 215. Using them will help MT students learn the fundamentals of proofreading and marking changes on an edited medical report. (*Note*: Not all the errors included would be caught by spell check. No student or practitioner should depend solely on spell check. Nothing takes the place of carefully proofreading your work.)

APPENDIX

1. Proofreader's marks

2. Challenging medical words, phrases, and prefixes

3. Lund Browder burn chart

4. Reference books and publishers

5. Healthcare Controlled Vocabulary

Challenging Medical Words, Phrases, and Prefixes

This list, developed over years of transcribing and teaching medical transcription students, represents some of the difficult words that trouble many healthcare workers and MTs. It is helpful to remove the list and keep at your workstation for quick referral, adding to the list as necessary.

Lund Browder Burn Chart

This is a standard burn chart used by many hospitals and burn centers, especially for pediatric burn patients. The Lund Browder chart shows the anterior and posterior aspects of the human body divided into segments. It is used to estimate the percentage of burned body tissue area. One of these charts is used on admission and at each debridement, which is a surgical procedure wherein both foreign material and contaminated tissue are removed, exposing healthy tissue. The Lund Browder chart is also used to show areas used as donor sites plus those areas covered with skin grafts and other types of grafts or dressings. This provides an ongoing picture of the progress in covering burn wounds. Published many years ago, this chart is widely used to help provide proper care for burn patients.

A Healthcare Controlled Vocabulary

The safety principles regarding language used by healthcare professionals, as described in this article by Dr. Neil Davis, are important for all MTs to understand. Dr. Davis is a pioneer in promoting these principles.

American Association for Medical Transcription

The American Association for Medical Transcription (AAMT) represents the medical transcription profession. AAMT has created a model job description, which is a practical, useful compilation of the basic job responsibilities of an MT.

AAMT defines an MT as a medical language specialist who interprets and transcribes dictation by physicians and other healthcare professionals regarding patient assessment, work-up, therapeutic procedures, clinical course, diagnosis, prognosis, etc., to document patient care and facilitate delivery of healthcare services.

AAMT MODEL JOB DESCRIPTION

Knowledge, Skills, and Abilities

1. Minimum education level of associate degree or its equivalent in work experience and continuing education

2. Knowledge of medical terminology, anatomy and physiology, clinical medicine, surgery, diagnostic tests, radiology, pathology, pharmacology, and the various medical specialties as required in areas of responsibility

3. Knowledge of medical transcription guidelines and practices

4. Excellent written and oral communication skills, including English usage, grammar, punctuation, and style

5. Ability to understand diverse accents and dialects and varying dictation styles

6. Ability to use designated reference materials

7. Ability to operate designated word processing, dictation, and transcription equipment, and other equipment as specified

8. Ability to work independently with minimal supervision

9. Ability to work under pressure with time constraints

10. Ability to concentrate

11. Excellent listening skills

12. Excellent eye, hand, an auditory coordination

13. Certified medical transcriptionist (CMT) status preferred

Working Conditions

General office environment
Quiet surroundings
Adequate lighting

Physical Demands

Primarily sedentary work with continuous use of earphones, keyboard, foot control, and, where applicable, video display terminal

Job Responsibilities

1. **Transcribes medical dictation to provide a permanent record of patient care.**

Performance Standards

1.1 Applies knowledge of medical terminology, anatomy and physiology, and English language rules to the transcription and proofreading of medical dictation from originators with various accents, dialects, and dictation styles.

1.2 Recognizes, interprets, and evaluates inconsistencies, discrepancies, and inaccuracies in medical dictation, and appropriately edits, revises, and clarifies them without altering the meaning of the dictation or changing the dictator's style.

1.3 Clarifies dictation that is clear or incomplete, seeking assistance as necessary.

1.4 Flags reports requiring the attention of the supervisor or dictator.

1.5 Uses reference materials appropriately and efficiently to facilitate the accuracy, clarity, and completeness of reports.

1.6 Meets quality and productivity standards and deadlines established by employer.

1.7 Verifies patient information for accuracy and completeness.

1.8 Formats reports according to established guidelines.

2. Demonstrates an understanding of the medicolegal implications and responsibilities related to the transcription of patient records to protect the patient and the business/institution.

Performance Standards

2.1 Understands and complies with policies and procedures related to medicolegal matters, including confidentiality, amendment of medical records, release of information, patients' rights, medical records as legal evidence, informed consent, etc.

2.2 Meets standards of professional and ethical conduct.

2.3 Recognizes and reports unusual circumstances and information with possible risk factors to appropriate risk management personnel.

2.4 Recognizes and reports problems, errors, and discrepancies in dictation and patient records to appropriate manager.

2.5 Consults appropriate personnel regarding dictation that may be regarded as unprofessional, frivolous, insulting, inflammatory, or inappropriate.

3. Operates designated word processing, dictation, and transcription equipment as directed to complete assignments.

Performance Standards

3.1 Uses designated equipment effectively, skillfully, and efficiently.

3.2 Maintains equipment and work area as directed.

3.3 Assesses condition of equipment and furnishings, and reports need for replacement or repair.

4. Follows policies and procedures to contribute to the efficiency of the medical transcription department.

Performance Standards

4.1 Demonstrates an understanding of policies, procedures, and priorities, seeking clarification as needed.

4.2 Reports to work on time, as scheduled, and is dependable and cooperative.

4.3 Organizes and prioritizes assigned work, and schedules time to accommodate work demands, turnaround-time requirements, and commitments.

4.4 Maintains required records, providing reports as scheduled and on request.

4.5 Participates in quality assurance programs.

4.6 Participates in evaluation and selection of equipment and furnishings.

4.7 Provides administrative/clerical/technical support as needed and as assigned.

5. Expands job-related knowledge and skills to improve performance and adjust to change.

Performance Standards

5.1 Participates in in-service and continuing education activities.

5.2 Provides documentation of in-service and continuing education activities.

5.3 Reviews trends and developments in medicine, English usage, technology, and transcription practices, and shares knowledge with colleagues.

5.4 Documents new and revised terminology, definitions, styles, and practices for reference and application.

5.5 Participates in the evaluation and selection of books, publications, and other reference materials.

6. Uses interpersonal skills effectively to build and maintain cooperative working relationships.

Performance Standards

6.1 Works and communicates in a positive and cooperative manner with management and supervisory staff, medical staff, coworkers and other healthcare personnel, and with patients with their families when providing information and services, seeking assistance and clarification, and resolving problems.

6.2 Contributes to team efforts.

6.3 Carries out assignments responsibly.

6.4 Participates in a positive and cooperative manner during staff meetings.

6.5 Handles difficult and sensitive situations tactfully.

6.6 Responds well to supervision.

6.7 Shares information with coworkers.

6.8 Assists with training of new employees as needed.[2]

AMERICAN ASSOCIATION FOR MEDICAL TRANSCRIPTION CODE OF ETHICS

Part I: Association Membership

Preamble

Be aware that it is by our standards of conduct and professionalism that the American Association for Medical Transcription (AAMT) is evaluated. As members of AAMT we should recognize and observe the goals and objectives of the organization and the limitations and confinements imposed by its bylaws, policies, and procedures.

Scope of Member Conduct

AAMT members (in individual categories of membership) will:

1. Place the goals and purposes of the Association above personal gain and work for the good of the profession.

2. Discharge honorably and to the best of their ability the responsibility of any elected or appointed Association position.

3. Preserve the confidential nature of professional judgments and determinations made confidentially by the official bodies of the Association.

4. Represent truthfully and accurately (a) one's membership in the Association, (b) one's roles and functions in the association, and (c) any positions and decisions of the association.

Part II: Professional Standards

Preamble

AAMT members are aware that it is by our standards of conduct and professionalism that the entire profession of medical transcription is evaluated. We should conduct ourselves in the practice of our professional so as to bring dignity and honor to ourselves and to the profession of medical transcription as medical language specialists. Therefore, the following standards are considered essential in the workplace:

1. A medical transcriptionist undertakes work only if s/he is competent to perform it.

2. A medical transcriptionist exhibits honesty and integrity in his/her professional work and activities.

3. A medical transcriptionist is reasonably familiar with and complies with principles of accuracy, authenticity, privacy, confidentiality, and security concerning patient care information.

4. A medical transcriptionist engages in professional reading and continuing education sufficient to stay abreast of important professional information.

5. A medical transcriptionist does not misrepresent or falsify information concerning medical records, his/her fees, work or professional experience, credentials, or affiliations.

6. A medical transcriptionist complies with applicable law and professional standards governing his/her work.

7. A medical transcriptionist does not assist others to violate ethical principles or professional standards of the medical transcription field.

8. If a medical transcriptionist learns of a significant unethical practice by another medical transcriptionist, s/he takes reasonable steps to resolve the matter.

9. A medical transcriptionist who agrees to serve in an official capacity in a professional association exhibits honesty and integrity in discharging his/her responsibilities.

[2]Copyright© 1990. Reprinted with permission of American Association for Medical Transcription, Modesto, CA.

10. AAMT members who are not medical transcriptionists should abide by the above principles where applicable.[3]

EMPLOYMENT AND CERTIFICATION POSSIBILITIES

Due to the variety of skills that MTs (medical language specialists) possess, they are employable in a variety of healthcare settings including doctors' offices, public and private hospitals, teaching hospitals, psychiatric hospitals, radiology departments, clinics, medical transcription services, pathology laboratories, insurance companies, medical libraries, government medical facilities, publishing companies, research facilities, and in the legal profession.

Experienced MTs may become teachers working in adult education to train future MTs. They may become reviewers, authors, or editors working through the publishing process to provide new and improved medical publications including course material and reference books.

Expert MTs who want to increase their professional responsibilities beyond medical transcription may become supervisors, managers, or owners of private transcription services.

After gaining experience as an MT, preferably in a hospital medical records department setting, one may apply to sit for the national medical certification examination sponsored by AAMT. A person who successfully completes the two-part examination earns the status of "Certified Medical Transcriptionist" (CMT), which is a mark of distinction in the field of medical transcription. A CMT is recognized as a dedicated, professional MT who participates in an ongoing program of continuing medical education approved by AAMT. CMTs are required to accrue 30 continuing education credit hours during a 3-year cycle to retain the CMT status.

For additional information about the medical transcription profession and the national certification examination, write the American Association for Medical Transcription, P.O. Box 576187, Modesto, CA 95357; or call 209/551-0883 or 800/982-2182. FAX 209/551-9317. E-mail aamt@sna.com

---

[3]Copyright 1995. Reprinted with permission of American Association for Medical Transcription, Modesto, CA.

Understanding Medical Records

Every time a patient enters Hillcrest Medical Center or Quali-Care Clinic—through the hospital admissions department, the hospital emergency room, for day surgery, or for outpatient treatment—a detailed record of the patient's care is created. Medical records are created by physicians and other healthcare providers dictating the results of their findings on patients they see, test, and examine. They originate patient reports that may be dictated in patient care areas, in pathology, radiology, other departments of the hospital, in the Clinic, or even off site. The hospital medical records are the property of Hillcrest Medical Center and are kept according to the regulations of the Joint Commission on Accreditation of Healthcare Organizations (JCAHO). Patients can get copies of their medical records; however, the information contained therein is confidential. No one has a right to obtain patient files without written permission (called an "authorization" or a "release") from the patient.

Certain circumstances require legal disclosure of confidential information to state departments of health or social services such as the following:

1. Birth and death

2. Blindness

3. Child abuse

4. Industrial poisoning

5. Vaccinations

6. Venereal and communicable diseases

7. Injuries resulting from criminal violence

8. Requests for plastic surgery without apparent reason (e.g., changing fingerprints or something that might indicate that the patient is a fugitive from justice)

Although laws vary from state to state relative to the length of time hospital medical records should be kept, both Hillcrest and Quali-Care Clinic chose to have each patient record microfilmed and retained for 25 years after the closure of the patient file. Because Hillcrest subscribes to voluntary accreditation by JCAHO, which means the hospital submits to inspections of each department by this agent of the federal government every 3 years and follows its guidelines, the medical records department is bound by JCAHO regulations in many of their departmental and record-keeping decisions.

The following eight basic medical reports are used at Hillcrest Medical Center.

1. History and Physical Examination Reports

2. Radiology Reports

3. Pathology Reports

4. Requests for Consultation

5. Operative Reports

6. Discharge Summaries

7. Death Summaries

8. Autopsy Reports

Examples of these documents are presented in the "Model Report Form" section, which begins on page 19. A brief explanation of each of these report forms follows. Additional tips for formatting your reports can be found in the "Transcription Using the Student Disk" section. The model report forms illustrate some of these guidelines.

HISTORY AND PHYSICAL EXAMINATION (H&P)

When a patient is admitted to the hospital for evaluation and treatment, the admitting/attending physician prepares a medical history detailing the specific complaint/illness that prompted admission to the hospital. Information about the patient's past medical history, surgery, allergies, and family and social histories, as well as psychiatric information may be included in this report. A review of the systems of the body (a survey of possible symptoms or historical facts relating to the patient's organs) may also be included. The content of the patient's history will vary depending on the chief complaint of the patient, on the physician's specialty, and on the physician's personal style; however, the history consists largely of subjective findings. The report of the physical examination includes vital signs and other objective findings by the physician.

The H&P is a priority item in the patient's hospital course because it is the summary of the information known at the time of admission. It should be dictated and transcribed within 24 hours of admission and, according to JCAHO and Hillcrest regulations, must be "charted" (placed in the medical record) before surgery can be accomplished. Model Report Form 1 on pages 19–20 displays a model report form for an H&P.

RADIOLOGY REPORT

Radiology is that branch of the health sciences dealing with radioactive substances and radiant energy together with the diagnosis and treatment of disease by means of roentgen rays (x-rays) or ultrasound techniques. The radiology report is a description of the findings and the interpretation of radiographs and other studies done by a radiologist.

Roentgenography is the making of a record of the internal structures of the body by passage of x-rays through the body to act on specially sensitized film. Special studies of the internal organs may require the use of contrast media (dyes) taken orally or by injection. Contrast media may be radiolucent (permitting the passage of roentgen rays) or radiopaque (not penetrable by roentgen rays or other forms of radiant energy). Ultrasonics deals with the frequency range beyond the upper limit of perception by the human ear. Ultrasound is used both therapeutically and as a diagnostic aid.

The numbering of these reports is done sequentially and includes the year performed. For example, a chest film from June 30, 1999 might be numbered 99-9062 to show that 9062 x-rays had been done by that date. Model Report Form 2 on page 21 shows a model radiology report.

OPERATIVE REPORT

Immediately after completion of a surgical procedure, a record of the procedure must be dictated by the physician, transcribed, and placed in the patient's file. This information is necessary for other physicians and allied health professionals who may be attending the patient. Preoperative and postoperative diagnoses are included. The body of the report (findings and procedures) is dictated in narrative form and contains information about the condition of the patient after surgery. See Model Report Form 3 on page 22 for a model operative report.

PATHOLOGY REPORT

Pathology is that branch of medicine dealing with the study of disease. It is divided into anatomic pathology and clinical pathology. Anatomic pathol-

ogy is the branch of pathology from which tissue reports are issued. The tissue is described both grossly and microscopically by a pathologist, a physician who determines the nature and extent of disease. The gross description of the tissue is done with the naked eye before the tissue is prepared for microscopic study. The microscopic description is done after the tissue has been specially prepared and mounted on a glass slide. It is carefully examined under a microscope, and a final diagnosis is issued. Special stains and other procedures, including consultations, are sometimes necessary to make a final diagnosis.

These reports are numbered sequentially and include the year performed and a letter to indicate autopsy (A), surgical pathology (S), or cytology report (C). For example, an autopsy done on June 30, 1999 might be numbered 99-A-25 to show that 25 autopsies had been done by that date. Model Report Form 4 on page 23 shows a model pathology report.

REQUEST FOR CONSULTATION

Consults from physicians specializing in different fields of medicine are necessary to provide proper care for the patient; however, the admitting/attending physician is in charge and maintains continuity of care at all times. For instance, when a patient is admitted to Hillcrest by a medical doctor who later determines that surgery may be necessary, the medical doctor often issues a request for consultation from a surgeon. The chosen surgeon answers this request by examining the patient and dictating a complete report of the examination, including a plan for treatment or surgery, and a prognosis. A model request for consultation form is shown in Model Report Form 5 on pages 24–25XX.

DISCHARGE SUMMARY

A discharge summary (also called a clinical résumé or final progress note) is required for each patient who is discharged from the hospital. It contains some of the same information that is included in the patient's admission history and physical examination. It also includes information about the admitting diagnosis, surgical procedures performed, laboratory and radiology studies, consultations, hospital course, the condition of the patient at the time of discharge, the medications prescribed on discharge, instructions for continuing care and therapy, prognosis, a discharge diagnosis, and possibly a date for a follow-up office visit. See Model

Report Form 6 on pages 26–27 for an example of a discharge summary.

DEATH SUMMARY

If a patient expires instead of being discharged from Hillcrest, a death summary is dictated. A death summary is a standard medical report <u>exactly like a discharge summary</u> but with some important, obvious differences.

The time and date of death, for example, must be recorded. Also included in the death summary might be whether or not the patient's family agreed to an autopsy, whether or not the patient was an organ donor, and whether or not the patient had a living will that called for no aggressive therapy, sometimes referred to as "do not resuscitate" or DNR status. Even if a patient does not have a living will, this decision is often made by the family or next of kin in an irreversible situation, and this information would be included in the death summary.

The cause of death may or may not be known when the death summary is dictated. At times, a pending surgical pathology report or autopsy report is needed before the cause of death can be confirmed. A model report form for a death summary is shown in Model Report Form 7 on pages 28–29.

AUTOPSY REPORT

An autopsy is done at Hillcrest only with permission from the relatives of the deceased unless the patient has died within 24 hours of admission, has died of an unknown cause, or has died under suspicious circumstances. If a patient case is determined to be medicolegal, that is, pertaining to medicine and the law (or to forensic medicine), the medical examiner or an appointed assistant is in charge of the disposition of the body. Nursing personnel, medical records personnel, and physicians on the staff of Hillcrest Medical Center are familiar with the requirements of the medical examiner's office.

The complete autopsy (or necropsy) report includes:

1. A preliminary diagnosis

2. A clinical history or brief résumé of the patient's medical history including the course in the hospital

3. The gross examination of the body, both external and internal, including evidence of injury

4. After the tissues removed at autopsy have been prepared, a microscopic description of the diseased organs is dictated along with the final diagnoses. Other special studies, opinions, or summary information may be included in the complete autopsy report depending on the specific nature of the case. See Model Report Form 8 on pages 30–35 for a model autopsy report.

OTHER MODEL REPORTS

Samples of HPIP (Model Report Form 9) and SOAP (Model Report Form 10) reports are also included on pages 36 and 37 of this section. These are reports used in the outpatient setting. They are discussed in detail on page 153, within the Quali-Care Clinic section. You will be using these models when you transcribe dictation exercises for the Quali-Care Clinic.

Model Report Forms

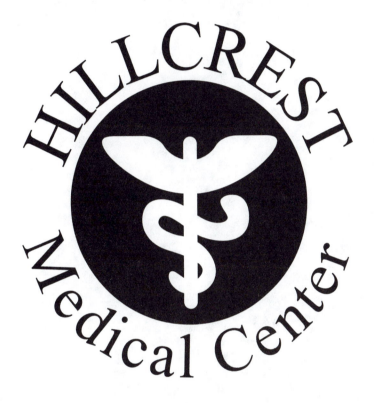

Model Report Form 1

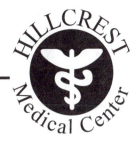

HISTORY AND PHYSICAL EXAMINATION (H&P)

Patient Name: Roger Parks ⟵———————————— 2 spaces after colons
2 spaces after periods
Hospital No.: 11009 No hyphenation
1-inch margins
Room No.: 812 Left justification

Date of Admission: 12/01/- - - - ⟵—— **Format date as MM/DD/YYYY**

Admitting Physician: Steven Benard, M.D.

Admitting Diagnosis: Rule out appendicitis.

CHIEF COMPLAINT: Abdominal pain.

HISTORY OF PRESENT ILLNESS: The patient is a 31-year-old white man with acute onset of right lower quadrant pain waking him up from sleep at approximately 3 a.m. on the morning of admission. The pain worsened throughout the day, radiating to his back and becoming associated with dry heaves. The patient states that the pain is constant and is worsened by walking or movement. The patient states his last bowel movement was on the previous evening and was normal. The patient is anorectic. He also gives a 1-year history of lower abdominal colicky pain associated with diarrhea. He was seen by his local medical doctor and given a diagnosis of irritable bowel syndrome; however, the pain is worse tonight and is unlike his previous bouts of abdominal pain. The patient also has had associated fever and chills to date.

PAST HISTORY: SURGICAL: No previous operations.
ILLNESSES: None. Hospitalization for epididymitis 10 years ago. He is ALLERGIC TO PENICILLIN. It makes him bloated. MEDICATIONS: None.

SOCIAL HISTORY: Carpenter. Lives with his wife and two children. He does not drink or smoke.

FAMILY HISTORY: Insignificant for familial inflammatory bowel disease except for the fact that his mother has colonic polyps. Father living and well. No siblings.

REVIEW OF SYSTEMS: Noncontributory.

PHYSICAL EXAMINATION: This is a 31-year-old white man with knees raised to his abdomen and complaining of severe pain. VITAL SIGNS: Admission temperature 99.6F; four hours after admission it was 102.6F. HEENT: Normocephalic, atraumatic, EOMs intact, negative icterus, conjunctivae pink. NECK: Supple. No adenopathy or bruits noted. CHEST: Clear to auscultation and percussion. CARDIAC: Regular rate and rhythm. No murmurs noted. Peripheral pulses 2+ and symmetrical. ABDOMEN: Bowel sounds initially positive but diminished. He has positive cough reflex, positive heel tap, and positive rebound tenderness. The pain is definitely worse in his RLQ. RECTAL: Heme negative. Tenderness toward the RLQ. Normal prostate. Normal male genitalia. EXTREMITIES: No clubbing, cyanosis, or edema. NEUROLOGIC: Nonfocal.

(Continued)

Use colons after brief introducers

HISTORY AND PHYSICAL EXAMINATION
Patient Name: Roger Parks
Hospital No.:   11009
Page 2

← Single space second and subsequent page heads

← Quadruple space between page header and text below (Text begins on fourth line following head)

LABORATORY DATA: Hemoglobin 14.6, hematocrit 43.6, and 13,000 WBCs. Sodium 138, potassium 3.8, chloride 105, CO_2 24, BUN 10, creatinine 0.9, and glucose 102. Amylase was 30. UA completely negative.

LFTs within normal limits. Alkaline phosphatase 78, GGT 9, SGOT 39, GPT 12, bilirubin 0.9. Flat plate and upright films of the abdomen revealed localized abnormal gas pattern in right lower quadrant. No evidence of free air.

ASSESSMENT: Rule out appendicitis. Some concern of whether this could be an exacerbation of developing inflammatory bowel disease. Due to the patient's history, increasing temperature, and localizing symptoms to his right lower quadrant, the patient needs surgical intervention to rule out appendicitis.

No extra space between dictator/transcriber initials

Quadruple space between last paragraph and signature rule →

_____
Steven Benard, M.D.

SB:xx
D:12/01/- - - -   **Format dates as**
T:12/01/- - - -   **MM/DD/YYYY**

Double space from signature block to dictator/transcriber initials

Align signature block with indent command at 4" position; signature rule is 25 underscores

Model Report Form 2

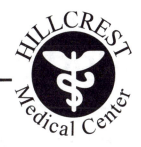

RADIOLOGY REPORT

Patient Name: Marietta Mosley

Hospital No.: 11446

X-ray No.: 98-2801

Admitting Physician: John Youngblood, M.D.

Procedure: Left hip x-ray.

Date: 08/05/- - - - ◄─── **Format date as MM/DD/YYYY**

PRIMARY DIAGNOSIS: Fractured left hip.

CLINICAL INFORMATION: Left hip pain. No known allergies.

Orthopedic device is noted transfixing the left femoral neck. I have no old films available for comparison. The left femoral neck region appears anatomically aligned. At the level of an orthopedic screw along the lateral aspect of the femoral neck, approximately at the level of the lesser trochanter, there is a radiolucent band consistent with a fracture of indeterminate age that shows probable nonunion. There is bilateral marginal sclerosis and moderate offset and angulation at this site.

◄─── **Double space between paragraphs**

Fairly exuberant callus formation is noted laterally along the femoral shaft.

IMPRESSION: 1. No evidence for significant displacement at the femoral neck.
Align text 2. Probable nonunion of fracture transversely through the shaft of the femur at about
using indent ─► the level of the lesser trochanter.
command

◄─── **Quadruple space between last paragraph and signature rule**

_____
Neil Nofsinger, M.D.

Use left justification and no hyphenation

Use 1-inch margins on side and bottom of report

Align signature block with indent command at 4" position; signature rule is 25 underscores

Double space between signature block and dictator/transcriber initials

Your initials

NN:xx
D:08/05/- - - -
T:08/05/- - - -

Model Report Form 3

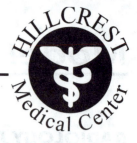

OPERATIVE REPORT

Patient Name: Kathy Sullivan

Hospital No.: 11525

Date of Surgery: 06/25/- - - -

Admitting Physician: Taylor Withers, M.D.

Surgeons: Sang Lee, M.D., Taylor Withers, M.D.

Preoperative Diagnosis: Urinary incontinence secondary to cystourethrocele.

Postoperative Diagnosis: Urinary incontinence secondary to cystourethrocele.

Operative Procedure: Total abdominal hysterectomy with Marshall-Marchetti correction.

Anesthesia: General endotracheal.

DESCRIPTION: After an abdominal hysterectomy had been performed by Dr. Withers, the peritoneum was closed by him and the procedure was turned over to me.

At this time the supravesical space was entered. The anterior portions of the bladder and urethra were dissected free by blunt and sharp dissection. Bleeders were clamped and electrocoagulated as they were encountered. A wedge of the overlying periosteum was taken and roughened with a bone rasp. The urethra was then attached to the overlying symphysis by placing two No. 1 catgut sutures on each side of the urethra and one in the bladder neck. The urethra and bladder neck pulled up to the overlying symphysis bone very easily with no tension on the sutures. Bleeding was controlled by pulling the bladder neck up to the bone. Penrose drains were placed on each side of the vesical gutter. Blood loss was negligible. The procedure was then turned back over to Dr. Withers, who proceeded with closure.

_____

Sang Lee, M.D.

SL:xx
D:06/25/- - - -
T:06/26/- - - -

Model Report Form 4

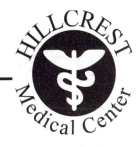

PATHOLOGY REPORT

Patient Name: Sumio Yukimura

Hospital No.: 11449

Pathology Report No.: 98-S-942

Admitting Physician: Donna Yates, M.D.

Preoperative Diagnosis: Cholelithiasis.

Postoperative Diagnosis: Cholelithiasis.

Specimen Submitted: Gallbladder and stone.

Date Received: 06/05/- - - -

Date Reported: 06/06/- - - -

GROSS DESCRIPTION: Specimen received in one container labeled "gallbladder." Specimen consists of a 9-cm gallbladder measuring 2 cm in average diameter. The serosal surface demonstrates diffuse fibrous adhesion. The wall is thickened and hemorrhagic. The mucosa is eroded, and there is a single large stone measuring 2 cm in diameter within the lumen. Representative sections are submitted in one cassette.

GROSS DIAGNOSIS: Gallstone.

KM:xx
D:06/05/- - - -
T:06/05/- - - -

Double space above and below sign-off blocks occurring between parts of a report

MICROSCOPIC DIAGNOSIS: Gallbladder, hemorrhagic chronic cholecystitis with cholelithiasis.

_____
Robert Thompson, M.D.

RT:xx
D:06/06/- - - -
T:06/06/- - - -

Model Report Form 5

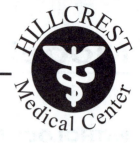

REQUEST FOR CONSULTATION

Patient Name: Marty Gibbs

Hospital No.: 11532

Consultant: Patrick O'Neill, M.D., Plastic Surgery

Requesting Physician: Diane Houston, M.D., Internal Medicine

Date: 11/25/- - - -

Reason for Consultation: Please evaluate extent of burn injuries.

BURNING AGENT: Coals in fire pit.

I have been asked to see this 5-year-old Caucasian male who appears in mild distress due to upper extremity burn after having fallen into hot coals in his back yard.

Using the Lund Browder chart,[4] the severity of burn is first and second degree. The total body surface area burned includes right lower arm 3%, right hand 1%. The joints involved include the right elbow, right wrist, right hand.

TREATMENT PLAN: Splinting right hand.

Use indent ⟶ Positioning: Elevation with splint on.
command to   Range of motion: Good mobility.
align text ↓   Pressure therapy: Will follow for induration, for pressure fracture.

GOALS: 1. Reduce risk of contractures of involved joints by positioning, splinting, and maintaining range of motion.
2. Reduce scar tissue formation by using Jobst bandages, pressure therapy, and splinting.
3. Obtain maximum mobility and strength of upper extremities.
4. Maximize independence in activities of daily living. Activity as tolerated.
5. Provide patient and family education regarding high-calorie, high-protein diet.

⟵ **Double space above**
   Continued notation

(Continued)

[4]See page xx: The Lund Browder Chart.

REQUEST FOR CONSULTATION   ← **Single space second and subsequent page heads**
Patient Name: Marty Gibbs
Hospital No.: 11532
Page 2

**Include at least 2 lines of
text on the top of a page
with a signature block**

↓

Thank you for asking me to see this delightful boy. I will follow him at the burn clinic in 2 weeks.

_____
Patrick O'Neill, M.D.

PO:xx
D:11/25/- - - -
T:11/28/- - - -

Model Report Form 6

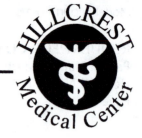

DISCHARGE SUMMARY

Patient Name: Joyce Mabry

Hospital No.: 11709

Admitted: 02/18/- - - -

Discharged: 02/24/- - - -

Consultations: Tom Moore, M.D., Hematology

Procedures: Splenectomy.

Complications: None.

Admitting Diagnosis: Elective splenectomy for idiopathic thrombocytopenic purpura and systemic lupus erythematosus.

HISTORY: The patient is a 21-year-old white woman who had noted excessive bruising since last June. She was diagnosed as having thrombocytopenic purpura. At the same time, the diagnosis of systemic lupus erythematosus was made. The patient continues with the bruising. The patient had been treated with steroids, prednisone 20 mg; however, the platelet count has remained low, less than 20,000. The patient was admitted for elective splenectomy.

LABORATORY DATA ON ADMISSION: Chest x-ray was negative. Electrocardiogram was normal. Sodium 138, potassium 5.2, chloride 104, CO_2 25, glucose 111. Urinalysis negative. Hemoglobin 14.8, hematocrit 43.5, white blood cell count 15,000, platelet count 17,000, PT 11.5, PTT 27.

HOSPITAL COURSE: The patient was taken to the operating room on February 19 where a splenectomy was performed. The patient's postoperative course was uncomplicated with the wound healing well. The platelet count was stable for the first 3 postoperative days. The patient was transfused intraoperatively with 10 units of platelets and postoperatively with 10 additional units of platelets. However, on the fourth postoperative day the platelet count had risen to 77,000, which was a significant increase.

The patient was discharged for follow-up in my office. She will also be seen by Dr. Moore, who will follow her SLE and ITP.

(Continued)

DISCHARGE SUMMARY
Patient Name: Joyce Mabry
Hospital No.: 11709
Page 2

DISCHARGE DIAGNOSIS: Idiopathic thrombocytopenic purpura and systemic lupus erythematosus.

DISCHARGE MEDICATIONS: 1. Prednisone 20 mg q.d.
                           2. Percocet 1 to 2 p.o. q. 4 h. p.r.n.
Use indent command ⟶ 3. Multivitamins, 1 in a.m. q.d.
to align text

_____
Carmen Garcia, M.D.

CG:xx
D:02/25/- - - -
T:02/26/- - - -

Model Report Form 7

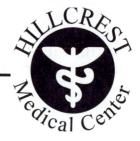

DEATH SUMMARY

Patient Name: Russell Syler

Hospital No.: 11663

Admitted: 05/15/- - - -

Deceased: 06/30/- - - -

Consultations: Hematology/Oncology.

Procedures: Abdominal ultrasound and insertion of Ommaya reservoir.

ADMITTING DIAGNOSES: Severe headache pain of 2 days' duration. Non-Hodgkin's lymphoma, large cell type.

FINAL DIAGNOSES:
1. Polymicrobial sepsis.
2. Nodular, diffuse, histiocytic lymphoma of head and neck with metastases to central nervous system and liver.
3. Pancytopenia secondary to chemotherapy and sepsis.
4. Bilateral pneumonia.
5. Urinary tract infection due to *Candida* organisms.
6. Oral herpes simplex viral infection.

COURSE IN HOSPITAL: This 33-year-old black man was originally admitted in early April with the diagnosis of nasopharyngeal mixed, nodular, histiocytic, diffuse, large-cell, noncleaved lymphoma with extensive involvement of the paranasal, parapharyngeal, and nasopharyngeal areas with erosion into the left orbit and cribriform plate and possible abdominal involvement. The patient required a tracheostomy secondary to stridor, status post radiation therapy to the neck and face in early May. He was status post chemotherapy with Cytoxan, adriamycin, vincristine, and prednisone every 3 weeks. His last chemotherapy had been administered 1 week prior to the current admission of May 15.

On admission the patient complained of intractable headache pain. He developed fever, chills, and sweats with nausea and vomiting, as well as decreased appetite for at least the past week. He also developed loose bowel movements on the day after admission. He had shortness of breath and a cough productive of yellow phlegm for the past week.

He had right upper quadrant and epigastric abdominal pain for the past week, not related to meals, with nausea and vomiting. He continued with positive frontal headache as well.

(Continued)

DEATH SUMMARY
Patient Name: Russell Syler
Hospital No.: 11663
Page 2

The patient's course deteriorated approximately 1 week into the hospital course with subsequent hypotension requiring dopamine for maintenance of blood pressure.

LABORATORY DATA: Blood cultures were positive for *Pseudomonas aeruginosa*. He was treated with tobramycin and penicillin G. As the sensitivity reports were returned from microbiology, vancomycin and Fortaz were added for better *Pseudomonas* coverage. Tobramycin was changed to amikacin when one of the patient's sputum cultures was positive for AFB, atypical, a slow grower, possible *Enterobacter* species. Two days prior to death, antituberculous medications, including INH and rifampin, were added, as well as amphotericin B for possible systemic fungal infection after urine cultures were positive for *Candida*. He was treated with a 5-day course of IV acyclovir for herpes simplex viral infection of the pharynx with resolution of the lesions.

The patient required multiple platelet transfusions as well as packed cells and occasional transfusions of fresh frozen plasma during his admission.

CAUSE OF DEATH: Secondary to circulatory collapse because of overwhelming sepsis, poor immune function, pancytopenia, and diffuse lymphomatous involvement. The patient's wife was notified of the grim prognosis and decided to make the patient "do not resuscitate" status.

The patient was pronounced dead on June 30, - - - -, at 4:12 a.m. Permission for autopsy was requested, but the family refused.

_____

Anthony Zanotti, M.D.

AZ:xx
D:07/03/- - - -
T:07/05/- - - -

Model Report Form 8

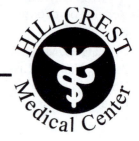

AUTOPSY REPORT

Patient Name: Wayne Kennedy

Hospital No.: 11509

Necropsy No.: 94-A-19

Admitting Physician: Joe Hernandez, M.D.

Pathologist: Loraine Muir, M.D.

Date of Death: 04/05/- - - -, 9 p.m.

Date of Autopsy: 04/06/- - - -, 8 a.m.

Admitting Diagnosis: Adenocarcinoma, maxilla.

Prosector: Keith Johnson, P.A.

FINAL ANATOMIC DIAGNOSES

1. Old fibrotic myocardial infarction of the anterior and septal walls of the left ventricle with anterior ventricular aneurysm, 4.5 x 3.0 cm.
2. Patchy old fibrotic myocardial infarction of the lateral and posterior septal walls of the left ventricle.
3. Probable recent ischemic changes, especially of the anterior and septal walls of the left ventricle.
4. Severe calcified atherosclerotic coronary vascular disease with up to 95% stenosis of the right coronary artery (RCA), up to 70% stenosis of the left anterior descending (LAD) coronary artery, and greater than 95% stenosis of the left circumflex coronary artery (LCCA).
5. Bilateral arterionephrosclerosis.
6. Atherosclerotic vascular disease, aorta, moderate to severe; circle of Willis, moderate.
7. Old infarct of right inner and inferior occipital lobe; small lacunar infarct, right caudate nucleus.
8. Bilateral pulmonary congestion, moderate.
9. Chronic passive congestion, liver, mild.
10. Simple cysts, right and left kidneys, up to 5.5 cm.
11. Diverticulum, 2.5 cm, duodenum.
12. Diverticulosis, sigmoid colon.
13. Status post partial left maxillectomy for adenocarcinoma, recent.

_____
Loraine Muir, M.D.

LM:xx
D:04/26/- - - -
T:04/26/- - - -

AUTOPSY REPORT
Patient Name: Wayne Kennedy
Hospital No.: 11509
Prosector: Keith Johnson, P.A.
Assistant: Yang Shen, P.A.

GROSS AUTOPSY EXAMINATION ← **Cap and center heads on autopsy report**

CLINICAL SUMMARY: Mr. Kennedy was a 74-year-old married Caucasian man who had been admitted to Hillcrest Medical Center on April 5 for re-resection of a left cheek mass, which had been resected in the past and was reported to be adenocarcinoma with margins involved. (See surgical report No. 98-S-125.) The patient's past medical history was remarkable for coronary artery disease, aortic stenosis, and angina. Past EKG reports revealed right bundle branch block, possible old anterior septal myocardial infarction, and probable ventricular aneurysm. Recent liver function studies were reported to be abnormal.

The patient underwent a partial left maxillectomy on the evening of April 5. The surgical procedure was uneventful, and the patient was sent to PAR in satisfactory condition at 7:55 p.m. However, shortly after his arrival in the recovery room, Mr. Kennedy suffered cardiopulmonary arrest. Code 19 was called at 8:12 p.m., and resuscitation efforts were begun immediately. Despite aggressive efforts, however, the patient was unable to be resuscitated and was pronounced dead at 9 p.m. on April 5.

AUTOPSY PERMISSION: Signed by the wife with no restrictions noted.

TIME AND DATE OF EXAMINATION: April 6, - - - -, 8 a.m.

VISITING PHYSICIANS: None.

EXTERNAL EXAMINATION: The body is that of an adult white man. The external appearance is consistent with the stated age. Total body length is 176 cm. Weight is estimated at 83 kg. The body is identified by a tag. Arterial embalming has not been performed. There is complete rigor mortis. There is posterior dependent lividity. There is moderate cyanosis of the nail beds of the fingers. Body heat and jaundice are absent. The nutritional status is adequate. The hair of the scalp is gray-brown with male pattern baldness. The irides are blue-gray, and the pupils measure 0.6 cm bilaterally. The skin surrounding the left eye has red-purple ecchymotic changes and appears slightly edematous. The sclera of the left eye is moderately congested. There is an 11.5-cm, recently sutured surgical incision beginning just superior to the central aspect of the upper lip and extending along the left side of the nose and beneath the left lower eyelid. An obturator and gauze packing are present in the area of the left maxilla with a portion of the maxilla having been recently surgically resected. An endotracheal tube is in place via the right naris. The ears are unremarkable. The neck is negative for abnormalities. The thoracic wall is normal in symmetry and anteroposterior diameter. A vascular catheter is present in the right subclavian region. The breasts are normal. The abdomen is concave. The external genitalia are normal male. A vascular catheter is present in the posterior aspect of the right hand. Two gold-colored bands are present on the fourth finger of the left hand. There is a rectangular 12.0 x 6.5 cm recent skin graft donor site on the anterior aspect of the left thigh. A 13.5 x 6.5 cm rectangular gray-tan to red, apparent previous skin graft donor site is present on the anterior aspect of the right leg. The posterior trunk is unremarkable. There are no palpable lymph nodes. There is no significant peripheral edema.

(Continued)

AUTOPSY REPORT
Patient Name: Wayne Kennedy
Hospital No.: 11509
Page 2

INCISIONS AND EVISCERATION: The trunk is opened with the usual Y-shaped incision. An intermastoid incision is used for examination of the brain. The organs of the trunk are removed using the Rokitansky method.

SUBCUTANEOUS TISSUE & MUSCLES: The subcutaneous fat of the midabdomen measures 3 cm in thickness and appears adequately hydrated. The skeletal musculature appears normal.

PERITONEAL CAVITY: The peritoneum is normal. The abdominal organs are normal in relation to each other. There is no increased fluid. There are no adhesions. The diaphragmatic leaves are normal. The inferior hepatic and splenic margins are normally located.

MEDIASTINUM & THYMUS: The mediastinum is of normal appearance with no shift of the trachea. The thymus is largely replaced by fat.

PLEURAL CAVITIES: There is no increased fluid. There are no adhesions.
PERICARDIAL CAVITY: There is no increased fluid. There are no adhesions.

HEART: The heart weighs 480 g and is normal in size, shape, and position. The epicardial surface is unremarkable. Serial sections through the coronary arteries reveal the proximal 3 cm of the right coronary artery to have approximately 40% to 70% focally calcific atherosclerotic stenosis. An irregular 4.0 x 0.3 x 0.2 cm, tan-red area of discoloration is present within the wall 2 cm from the origin. The subsequent 1.3 cm of the right coronary artery has greater than 95% stenosis with severe calcification. The remainder of this artery has approximately 20% to 30% stenosis. The left anterior descending and left circumflex coronary arteries each have separate ostia arising behind the left cusp of the aortic valve. Each of these ostia is widely patent. The left anterior descending coronary artery has approximately 40% to 60% calcific atherosclerotic stenosis throughout its length. The first 2.5 cm of the circumflex coronary artery has approximately 60% to 75% calcific atherosclerotic stenosis. A subsequent 0.7-cm segment has tan-red to gray thrombus material filling its lumen. The subsequent 0.7 cm of this artery has approximately 50% stenosis. Following this is a 1-cm segment, which is occluded by gray to tan rubbery thrombus material. The remainder of the artery has approximately 40% to 60% stenosis. A right dominant coronary arterial system is present. The atria measure 0.2 cm in thickness and are normal in appearance. The foramen ovale is closed. The right ventricle measures 0.3 cm in thickness. The left ventricle measures 1.5 cm in thickness just inferior to the mitral annulus. There is a 4.5 x 3.0 cm soft aneurysmic dilatation of the central anterior wall of the left ventricle. The anterior wall has transmural gray-white rubbery fibrotic changes extending from the apex to the central aspect. The wall of this area ranges in thickness from 0.2 cm to 0.5 cm. There are circumferential rubbery gray-white fibrotic changes of the apical myocardium of the left ventricle and transmural, similar fibrotic changes of the septum extending from the apex to the central portion. In the areas of greatest fibrosis, the septum measures only 0.3 cm in thickness. Patchy fibrotic changes are present throughout the left half of the remainder of the septal wall extending to the base. There is slight extension of the fibrotic changes to the left lateral ventricular wall at the base. There are no mural thrombi. The endocardium of the

(Continued)

AUTOPSY REPORT
Patient Name: Wayne Kennedy
Hospital No.: 11509
Page 3

aneurysmal area has focal firm gray-tan apparent calcification, the largest area of which measures 0.1 cm in greatest dimension. The valves of the heart measure 14, 10, 11, and 7 cm for the tricuspid, pulmonic, mitral, and aortic, respectively. There is a slight rubbery thickening of the cusps of the aortic valve, but otherwise the valves are grossly unremarkable. The chordae tendineae and the trabecular muscle of the right ventricle are multiple, thin, threadlike fibrous bands that measure less than 0.1 cm in thickness and up to 4.5 cm in length. These bands form a spiderweb-like meshwork within the right ventricular cavity at the base.

GREAT VESSELS: The main pulmonary arteries contain neither emboli nor atherosclerotic plaque. The ductus arteriosus is closed. The aorta has moderate to severe calcific atherosclerosis with scattered areas of intimal ulceration measuring up to 2 cm in greatest dimension. The ostium of the right renal artery has approximately 75% stenosis; the ostium of the left renal artery is widely patent. Both arteries have mild to moderate atherosclerotic plaque.

THYROID: This gland is normal in shape, size, color, and consistency.

PARATHYROIDS: No enlargement of these glands is demonstrable.

LARYNX & TRACHEA: The larynx and trachea are normal. There is no hyperemia of the mucosa.

LUNGS & BRONCHI: The right lung weighs 520 g. The left lung weighs 420 g. The pleural surface of each is reddish pink to dark red with mild to moderate anthracotic pigmentation. The smaller pulmonary arteries contain no emboli or significant atherosclerotic change. The bronchi contain a small amount of reddish tan, mucoid-appearing material, and the bronchial mucosa is mildly hyperemic. The parenchyma of the lower lobes and dependent portions of each lung have a moderate, dark red, congested appearance. The cut surface exudes a small amount of frothy pink-red fluid. There is an 0.6 x 0.5 x 0.5 cm, tan, finely granular calcified area within the parenchyma of the left lower lobe. No other focal lesions are identified. A lymph node near the hilum of the right lung has an 0.5 cm, firm, calcified, gray granulomatous-appearing area.

GASTROINTESTINAL TRACT: The esophagus is normal with no significant degree of leukoplakia. The serosa of the stomach is smooth and glistening. The stomach contains a small quantity of fluid material. The mucosa of the stomach has the usual rugal pattern. There are no ulcerations, erosions, or tumors of the gastric mucosa. The pylorus is normal. There is a 2.5 x 1.5 x 1.5 cm diverticulum of the wall of the duodenum 8 cm distal to the pyloric sphincter. The ampulla of Vater enters into the proximal side of this diverticulum. The duodenum is otherwise unremarkable. The small intestine contains a small amount of liquid material. The mucosa of the small intestine is normal. The cecum contains a moderate amount of brown semiliquid stool. The mucosa of the colon is examined in its entirety and found to be normal. No polyps, tumors, diverticula, or ulcers are noted. The vermiform appendix is unremarkable. The omentum is normal, as are the mesenteric arteries, veins, and fat.

LIVER: The liver weighs 1920 g. The capsule is smooth and glistening with no evidence of thickening. The sectioned surface reveals a normal hepatic parenchyma with no accentuation of the lobular pattern. There are no scars or nodules. The parenchyma is dry and reddish tan. The portal vein and the hepatic artery are normal.

(Continued)

AUTOPSY REPORT
Patient Name: Wayne Kennedy
Hospital No.: 11509
Page 4

GALLBLADDER: The gallbladder is normal in location, shape, and size and is free of adhesions. It contains a moderate amount of thick, dark green viscid bile. No calculi are present. There are no papillomas of the mucosa, and there is no cholesterolosis. The cystic duct is normal. The common bile duct is somewhat dilated, measuring 2 cm in circumference, but is lined by the usual velvety epithelium. No areas of obstruction are identified.

PANCREAS: The peripancreatic fat is normal. The pancreas is serially sectioned revealing a normal, pale tan, firm consistency. There are no tumor nodules. The pancreatic duct is not distended, and the blood vessels are normal.

SPLEEN: The spleen weighs 140 g. The capsule is smooth and opaque. There are no areas of fibrosis. The sectioned surfaces show no accentuation of the malpighian bodies or trabeculations. The interior of the spleen is dark red and firm.
ADRENALS: These glands are normal in size, shape, consistency, and position. The cortices are a vivid yellow and no nodules are present. The medullae are gray with no nodules.

KIDNEYS: The right kidney weighs 200 g, and the left kidney weighs 210 g. The capsules appear normal and strip with ease. The underlying renal surfaces are dark red and coarsely granular. A large 5.5 cm, smooth-walled cyst filled with straw-colored serous fluid is present in the peripheral cortex of the upper pole of the left kidney. Two similar cysts measuring 3.5 and 2.5 cm in diameter are present within the cortex of the lower pole and central lateral aspect of the right kidney, respectively. The cortices of each kidney range in thickness from 0.4 cm to 0.7 cm. The medullae appear normal. The corticomedullary junctions are mildly indistinct. There are no tumors, infarcts, or areas of scarring. The calyces and pelves are not dilated. The mucosa is normal. The arteries and veins appear normal. The perirenal fat is unremarkable.

URETERS & BLADDER: The ureters are patent throughout with no dilatations or obstructions. The urinary bladder contains a small amount of yellow urine. The walls of the bladder are of normal thickness, and the mucosa is moderately trabeculated. No calculi are present within the urinary tract.

GENITAL ORGANS: The prostate is located in the usual position and is normal in size. The parenchyma has the usual gray-pink appearance and rubbery consistency with mild to moderate nodularity. There is no obstruction to the urinary outflow tract. The seminal vesicles are unremarkable. The testicles are normal by palpation.

LYMPH NODES: The right hilar lymph node has the previously described granulomatous area present. Similar, firm, calcified, gray, granulomatous areas are present within two mediastinal lymph nodes, the largest of these granulomatous areas measuring 1.5 cm in greatest dimension. The cervical, periaortic, iliac, mesenteric, omental, and axillary nodes are unremarkable.

BONES & JOINTS: The cartilage at the sternoclavicular joint is slightly more prominent than usual. The joints otherwise are unremarkable.

(Continued)

AUTOPSY REPORT
Patient Name: Wayne Kennedy
Hospital No.: 11509
Page 5

BONE MARROW: Vertebral marrow from the lumbar area and from the ribs appears grossly normal.

CRANIAL CAVITY: There is no evidence of recent or old skull fractures, epidural or subdural hemorrhages. There is no focal or diffuse thickening of the skull cap.

BRAIN: The leptomeninges covering the brain are translucent and thin. The brain weighs 1480 g. The gyri and sulci of the cerebral cortex are normal. There are no pressure ridges on the uncinate gyri, and there is no coning of the cerebellum. The vessels comprising the circle of Willis show no abnormalities. No aneurysms are present. There is moderate atherosclerosis. The brain will undergo further fixation in a 10% formalin solution and will be further described at Neuropathology Conference.

_____
Loraine Muir, M.D.

LM:xx
D:04/06/- - - -
T:04/10/- - - -   ←—————— **Double space between
                                 transcribed date and copy line**

C: Joe Hernandez, M.D.

Model Report Form 9

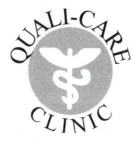

History, Physical, Impression, Plan (HPIP)

Patient Name: Margaret Thornton   PCP: R. J. Reardon, M.D.
Date of Birth: 4/7/- - - -   Age: 27   Sex: Female
Date of Exam: 9/23/- - - -

← **Double space here and between paragraphs**

HISTORY OF PRESENT ILLNESS: Fever and some cough since 9/20/- - - - when she was started on
Biaxin 500 mg, 1 p.o. b.i.d. Fever has continued since that time at 101.5F, taken orally as soon as her
Tylenol wears off. No current *Pneumocystis* prophylaxis; says that her T-cell count was 86 last time. She
complains of headaches but denies changes in vision. She has right-sided chest pain, particularly by the
end of the day and with movement.

MEDICATIONS: Mycostatin suspension, multivitamins, Elavil 10 mg p.r.n., Ativan 1 mg b.i.d. p.r.n., the
Biaxin, and Diflucan 200 mg, 1 p.o. b.i.d. Only a 2-day supply of Diflucan was given.

LAB DATA: WBC count of 5500 with differential 42% neutrophils, 34% lymphocytes, 9% monocytes, and
3% eosinophils. Hematocrit 44%, platelets 199,000. Chest x-ray: Mild interstitial looking fuzziness bilaterally, more on right than on left.

PHYSICAL EXAMINATION: In general a chronically ill white female, weight down 2 lb. since her last
visit, energy level is down. HEENT: Oral cavity erythematous, no thrush. NECK: A few small cervical
lymph nodes are palpated. CHEST: Mild decreased breath sounds on the right but no frank rales or
rhonchi. No murmurs or rubs. SKIN is clear; no signs of herpes zoster reactivation. Face is somewhat
flushed. ABDOMEN is scaphoid with bowel sounds present in all four quadrants. EXTREMITIES: Some
mild peripheral neuropathy bilaterally; reflexes and pulses intact bilaterally.

IMPRESSION: AIDS with progression of disease.

PLAN: We had a long talk regarding her medication, her T-cell count, the possibility that she has had a progression in her disease, and that she would need to slow down. She is to be off work for this week, and we
will see her back here next week.

_____
Robert Solenberger, M.D.
Infectious Disease

RS:xx
D:9/23/- - - -
T:9/24/- - - -

Model Report Form 10

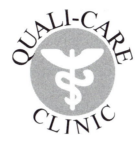

Subjective, Objective, Assessment, Plan (SOAP)

Patient Name: Mitchell Fitzpatrick
Date of Birth: 6/17/- - - -   Age: 53
Date of Exam: 2/1/- - - -

PCP: Norma Jacobs, M.D.
Sex: Male

SUBJECTIVE: Mr. Fitzpatrick presents for follow-up of his hemoptysis, which has improved significantly. He underwent flexible fiberoptic bronchoscopy as an outpatient at Hillcrest on 1/27/- - - - with no endobronchial abnormalities noted. It is suspected, therefore, that his expectoration of blood is not coming from his lungs. The patient has had worsening dyspnea on exertion, according to his wife, with several episodes of nocturnal wheezing associated with mild shortness of breath.

Use indent feature for these paragraphs, single spaced ⟶ ↕

OBJECTIVE: Spirometry shows an FEV_1 of 2.59, 82% of predicted. His FEV_1 to FVC ratio is 79%. FVC is 3.26, 71% of predicted. There is mild reduction in the midflow rates. On exam, oropharynx is clear. Neck is supple without adenopathy or bruits. Lung fields are clear to auscultation. Cardiac exam: Regular rate and rhythm with a soft systolic murmur heard best at the right upper sternal border and left apex. No significant peripheral edema or cyanosis.

ASSESSMENT
1. Hemoptysis, no evidence of endobronchial lesions.
2. Obesity.
3. Probable bronchospastic lung disease.
4. History of hypertension, remote.
5. History of peptic ulcer disease, remote.

PLAN
1. We will start the patient empirically on an Albuterol inhaler, two puffs q.4 h. p.r.n. wheezing or dyspnea.
2. He will be instructed on the proper use of his inhaler.
3. Follow-up in 4 months for repeat spirometry testing.

Gerald Warr Wells, M.D.
Pulmonology

GWW:xx
D:2/1/- - - -
T:2/2/- - - -

References

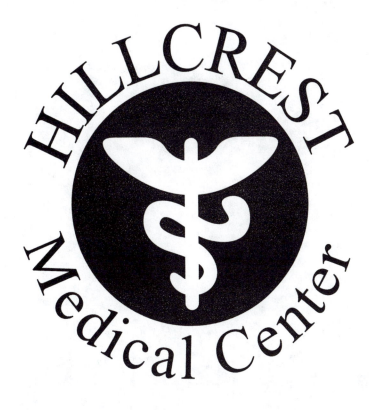

Transcription Rules for Hillcrest Medical Center and Quali-Care Clinic

Each hospital has a process by which the abbreviations and style for its transcribed medical records are set. This process usually involves the Medical Records Committee (comprised of appointed members of the medical staff) together with representatives from both the medical records department and hospital administration. The rules adopted for medical reports at Hillcrest have been voluntarily adopted for use at Quali-Care Clinic, and they include the following:

CAPITALIZATION

1. Use initial capital letters in eponymic terms. Eponyms are names of phrases formed from or including the name of a person. The common noun following the eponym is lowercase.

   Examples:

   Rocky-Davis incision

   Foley catheter

   Down's syndrome

   May-Hegglin anomaly

   Duffy blood group

   Crohn's disease

   NOTE:

   Some reference books show the possessive and some do not. At Hillcrest, *Dorland's Illustrated Medical Dictionary* and *Stedman's Medical Dictionary* are our preferred medical references, and we accept their styling of eponymic terms.

2. Capitalize trade names and proprietary names of drugs and brand names of manufactured products and equipment. Do **not** capitalize generic names or descriptive terms.

   Examples:

   Trade names of drugs include Keflex, Motrin, and Bayer. Corresponding generic terms are cephalaxin, ibuprofen, and aspirin.

   Trade names of suture materials include Vicryl, Dexon, and Prolene. Generic terms include chromic catgut, silk, nylon, and cotton—either plain, braided, or twisted.

   Miscellaneous brand names include Kleenex, Vaseline, and Scotch tape. Corresponding generic terms are tissue, petroleum jelly, and cellophane tape.

3. Use an initial capital letter and italics (or underscore to indicate italics) for the name of a genus when used in the singular. Do not capitalize, italicize, or underscore when used in the plural or as an adjective. Names of species are lowercase and are italicized or underscored when used with the genus name. After first mention, the genus name may be referred to by the initial—some reference books use a period and some do not—with the species name following.

   Examples:

   Pseudomonas aeruginosa

   (P aeruginosa)

   Staphylococcus aureus

   (S aureus)

   BUT

   pseudomonal appearing

   staphylococcal organism

4. Departmental names within Hillcrest Medical Center are lowercase.

Examples:

operating room

postanesthesia recovery

blood bank

transcription section

5. Capitalize the proper names of languages, races, religions, and sects. Do **not** capitalize the common nouns following these designations. Do **not** capitalize informal designations of race, i.e., white or black.

Examples:

Asians

Hispanic people

the English language

of Jewish ancestry

African-Americans

Seminoles

6. As a courtesy, positive allergy information may be either underscored or keyed in all capital letters in order to call attention to this vital information.

Example:

ALLERGIES: The patient is allergic to SULFA.

7. Capitalize acronyms but not the words from which the acronym is derived.

Examples:

nonsteroidal anti-inflammatory drug (NSAID)

coronary artery bypass graft (CABG)

magnetic resonance imaging (MRI)

NUMBERS

1. Spell the numbers "one" through "nine" when they appear in a narrative section of a medical report. When one numerical expression follows another, for clarity, spell out the one that can more easily be expressed in words.

Examples:

Dr. Smith removed seven lesions from the patient's back and three from his right leg.

The dietician recommended two 6-ounce cans of supplement daily.

2. Use figures with technical information, i.e., in laboratory results, vital signs, age, height, weight, drug dosages.

Examples:

Apgar scores were 9/9 at 1 and 5 minutes respectively.

Lipoproteins included an LDL of 80 and an HDL of 50.

Vital signs showed blood pressure 120/80, pulse 72/minute and regular, respirations 21, temperature 98 degrees F.

Medications: Lomotil 20 mg at bedtime, diazepam 15 mg daily.

3. Always use figures with abbreviations, symbols, and measurements—no space comes between the number and its symbol, but use one space between otherwise.

Examples:

Pulses 2+, 100% oxygen, 15 mm Hg, reflexes 5/5 throughout

The uterus weighs 150 g and measures 8.0 x 4.5 x 0.9.

NOTE:

In the measurement above, while the whole number has a zero added for balance, the final measurement has a preceding zero added for clarity. **The preceding zero is mandatory in decimal phrases.**

4. A space should appear between an arabic number and the corresponding unit of measure abbreviation/symbol.

Examples:

9 mg%, 83 mL, 0.5 cm, 64 g/dL

5. Spell out ordinal numbers **except** when a date is used with the month.

Examples:

An incision was made between the fifth and sixth ribs. (**not** 5th and 6th)

The patient had a seventh nerve palsy. (**not** 7th and **not** VIIth)

A Foley catheter was inserted the third day after surgery.

(**BUT** On October 3, surgery was performed.

6. Numbers that constitute a series or range should be written as figures if at least one of them is greater than nine or is a mixed or decimal fraction. When indicating a span of years or page numbers do **not** omit digits.

Examples:

The gallstones measured 0.5, 1.2, and 3.7 cm, respectively.

Statistics proved the theory in 8 of 12 recipients.

The patient took epilepsy medication from 1990 to 1993. (**not** 1990-93)

The solution can be found on pages 157 to 159. (**not** 157-159)

NOTE:

The use of a hyphen in a span of years or page numbers is discouraged because of the confusion about whether it should be read as "to" or "through."

7. The vertebral or spinal column segments are referred to in arabic numerals. The 12 pairs of cranial nerves, however, are referred to in roman numerals.

Examples:

cervical spine = C1 through C7

thoracic spine = T1 through T12

dorsal spine = D1 through D12 (interchangeable with thoracic spine)

lumbar spine = L1 through L5

sacral spine = S1 through S5

BUT cranial nerves I through XII

8. Titers and ratios are expressed with figures and a colon. The colon is read as "to."

Examples:

Cord blood showed a herpes titer of 1:110.

Anesthesia consisted of Xylocaine and epinephrine 1:100,000.

9. Temperature readings are expressed in either Celsius (C) or Fahrenheit (F). At Hillcrest, the symbol for the word "degrees" is not used.

Each of the following examples is acceptable:

98.6F or 98.6 degrees F or 98.6 degrees Fahrenheit

35.4C or 35.4 degrees C or 35.4 degrees Celsius

10. Stainless and nonstainless steel sutures are sized by the United States Pharmacopeia (USP) system. Sizes range from 11-0 (smallest) to 7 (largest). Sizes No. 1 through No. 7 are expressed as whole numbers. Stainless steel suture sizes may also be sized by the Brown and Sharp (B&S) gauge. B&S sizes are expressed in whole numbers from No. 40 (smallest) to No. 20 (largest).

Examples:

Then 9-0 silk was used for the eye wounds.

The peritoneum was closed with 3-0 chromic catgut.

No. 5 wire was used for the skin.

NOTE:

In the example above, No. 5 is the preferred style for Hillcrest, though #5 is seen in some reference material.

11. Superscripts and subscripts are used in medical dictation; however, if the transcription equipment being used does not provide for entering characters either above or below the line, the superscript and/or subscript may be entered on the line. In either case, no spaces should be used.

Examples:

H2O or H_2O		PO2 or PO_2
^{131}I	**BUT**	I 131
^{198}Au	**BUT**	Au 198

12. Use arabic numerals when referring to EKG leads, cancer grades, and both conventional and military time.

Examples:

EKG leads V1 to V6　　grade 2 tumor

1600 hours is 4 p.m.

NOTE:

When time on a clock is used to describe a location, use the following style:

Suspicious area tagged with a suture at 3 o'clock.

Lesions identified at 12, 3, and 6 o'clock.

PUNCTUATION

Apostrophe

1. The apostrophe is used to show possession.

   Examples:

   Patient's condition (singular possessive noun)

   Doctors' opinion (plural possessive noun)

2. The apostrophe is used to form contractions.

   Examples:

   He's having no symptoms. (contraction of he is)

   It's my opinion. (contraction of it is)

   BUT

   Its measurements are irregular. (possessive pronoun—no apostrophe used here)

3. Do **not** use an apostrophe to form the plural of either an all-capital abbreviation or of numerals, including years.

   Examples:

DRGs	Temperature in the 20s
WBCs	Born in the 1990s
D&Cs	Three Ph.D.s attended

   NOTE:

   When a word or letter could be misread, the apostrophe is sometimes used for clarity.

   Examples:

   He received all A's.　　The T's were left uncrossed.

Her U's need work.　　Record the patient's I's and O's.

4. The apostrophe is used with units of time and money used as possessive adjectives.

   Examples:

   a week's work/a dollar's work/in a month's time (all show singular possessive)

   seven days' work/50 cents' worth/six months' gestation (all show plural possessive)

Hyphen

1. Hyphenate a compound in which a number is the first element and the compound precedes the noun it modifies.

   Examples:

   48-hour turnaround　　a 12-factor panel

   a 5-g cyst　　two 6-in. lacerations

2. Hyphenate a compound adjectival phrase when it precedes the noun it modifies, but **not** when it is in the predicate.

   Examples:

   a 17-week infant (The infant was 17 weeks old.)

   end-to-end anastomosis (The anastomosis was end to end.)

   a figure-of-eight suture (The suture was in a figure of eight.)

3. Hyphenate an adjective-noun compound when it precedes and modifies another noun.

   Examples:

   upper-range results (The results were in the upper range.)

   third-floor burn unit (The burn unit was on the third floor.)

4. Hyphenate two or more adjectives used coordinately or as conflicting terms whether they precede the noun or follow as a predicate adjective.

   Examples:

   false-positive results (The results were false-positive.)

double-blind study (The study was done as a double-blind.)

5. Hyphenate color terms when the two elements are of equal weight.

    Examples:

    pink-tan tissue   gray-brown area

    BUT

    pinkish tan mucosa   grayish brown skin

6. When expressing numbers in words, hyphenate all compound numbers between 21 and 99, either ordinal or cardinal numbers. Also, use a hyphen when expressing fractions in words.

    Examples:

    thirty-five miles later

    one hundred forty-five

    left one-third empty

    three-fourths agreed

7. Use a hyphen when joining numbers or letters to form a word, phrase, or abbreviation.

    Examples:

    5-FU   C-section   X-ray   T-spine

    VP-16   SMA-12   Y-shaped incision

ABBREVIATIONS AND SYMBOLS

Abbreviations

Abbreviations used in Hillcrest Medical Center case studies are listed and defined in the medical terminology glossary preceding each case. They are also listed alphabetically in the index.

"Abbreviations are a convenience, a time saver, a space saver, and a way of avoiding the possibility of misspelling words. However, a price can be paid for their use. Abbreviations are sometimes not understood, misread, or are interpreted incorrectly. Their use may lengthen the time needed to train individuals in the health fields, wastes the time of healthcare workers in tracking down their meaning, at times delays the patient's care, and occasionally results in patient harm.

Healthcare organizations are wisely required by the Joint Commission on Accreditation of Healthcare

Organizations to formulate an approved list of abbreviations. Every attempt should be made to restrict this list to common abbreviations that are understood by all health professionals who must work with medical records."[5]

The information presented in both the heading of each Hillcrest medical report and, at times, in the body of the report will be in what is known as elliptical or "clipped" expressions, i.e., a word or words that represent a complete thought. These "clipped" expressions are commonly used in medical dictation and each will end with a period to show they are complete thoughts. *NOTE: Hillcrest medical records will have no abbreviations used in the diagnosis lines, impression lines, preoperative or postoperative lines.*

Symbols

1. The virgule (slash or diagonal) is used to indicate the word "per" in laboratory values and other equations or the word "over" in blood pressure (BP) readings and visual acuity.

    Examples:

    using the virgule for "per"

    hemoglobin 14.1 g/dL

    fasting blood sugar 138 mg/dL

    using the virgule for "over"

    blood pressure 110/70 mm Hg in both arms

    20/80 right eye and 20/40 left eye (visual acuity)

    NOTE: Referring to the first BP example above, if millimeters of mercury is dictated, mm Hg is transcribed. If, however, this phrase is not dictated, it may be omitted. Millimeters of mercury can be used in recording either ocular tension or blood pressure readings.

2. Lowercase "x" is used to indicate "by" in measurements and to indicate "times" in magnification and multiplication.

    Examples:

    Sponge and instrument count was correct x 3. (x = times)

[5]Published with permission from *Medical Abbreviations: 12,000 Conveniences at the Expense of Communications and Safety*, 8th edition, 1997, published by Neil M. Davis Associates, Huntingdon Valley, Pennsylvania 19006.

Fetal limb length was 5.5 x 1.5 x 1.0 cm. (x = by)

Electron microscopy cells magnified x 100,000. (x = times)

3. Use numerals with a symbol or an abbreviation. When the phrase is spelled out, however, spell out the numbers as well.

Examples:

Deep tendon reflexes two plus (not two +)

OR

Deep tendon reflexes 2+ (not 2 plus)

4. Both reflexes and pulses are usually graded on a scale from zero to four plus. The meanings of the different grades are as follows:

Reflexes

4+ = very brisk, hyperactive; may indicate disease; often associated with clonus (alternating muscular contraction and relaxation in rapid succession)

3+ = brisker than average; possibly but not necessarily indicative of disease

2+ = average or normal

1+ = somewhat diminished; low normal

0 = no response; may indicate neuropathy

Pulses

0 = completely absent

+1 = markedly impaired

+2 = moderately impaired

+3 = slightly impaired

+4 = normal

5. Qualitative test results are usually given using the plus and minus symbols.

Examples:

– negative

+/– very slight trace or reaction

+ slight trace or reaction

++ trace or noticeable reaction

+++ moderate amount of reaction

++++ large amount of pronounced reaction

6. The metric system of measurement is used in medicine. (See the list that follows.) Use the abbreviated forms when entering number, with metric measurements. Do not use a period following metric abbreviations. Do not pluralize abbreviations. (Liter is abbreviated with an uppercase L.)

Examples:

1 cm	0.9 cm	20 cm
1 mL	1.6 mL	15 mL
1 g	3.7 g	32 g
1 L	2.5 L	8 L

7. Latin abbreviations: At Hillcrest these are keyed in lowercase with periods, as follows:

a.c. (ante cibum, before meals)

a.d. (auris dextra, right ear)

a.m. (ante meridiem, morning)

a.s. (auris sinistra, left ear)

a.u. (auris utraque, each ear)

b.i.d. (bis in die, twice a day)

d. (die, day)

h. (hour)

h.s. (hora somni, bedtime)

n.p.o (nil per os, nothing by mouth)

o.d. (oculus dexter, right eye)

o.s. (oculus sinister, left eye)

o.u. (oculus uterque, each eye)

p.c. (post cibum, after meals)

p.m. (post meridiem, afternoon)

p.o. (per os, by mouth)

p.r.n. (pro re nata, as circumstances may require)

q.d. (quaque die, every day)

q.h. (quaque hora, every hour)

q.i.d. (quater in die, four times a day)

q.l. (quantum libet, as much as desired)

q.p. (quantum placeat, as much as desired)

q.s. (quantum satis, sufficient quantity)

t.i.d. (ter in die, three times a day)

LIST OF METRIC MEASUREMENTS

Unit	Abbreviation
centimeter(s)	cm
cubic centimeter(s)	cc or cm^3
cubic meter(s)	m^3
deciliter(s)	dL
gram(s)	g
kilocalorie(s)	kcal
kilogram(s)	kg
kiloliter(s)	kL
kilometer(s)	km
liter(s)	L
meter(s)	m
microgram(s)	mcg
milligram(s)	mg
milliliter(s)	mL
millimeter(s)	mm
square centimeter(s)	sq cm or cm^2
square kilometer(s)	sq km or km^2
square meter(s)	sq m or m^2

CMTips™

DIFFICULT SINGULAR/PLURAL WORDS AND PHRASES

These have proven to be difficult because we cannot rely on their being dictated correctly. *Beware* and transcribe as follows:

Singular	Plural
ala nasi is	alae nasi are
diverticulum is	diverticula are
genitalis is	genitalia are
naris is	nares are
medium is	media are
labium	labia
majus is	majora are
minus is	minora are
lentigo is	lentigines are
focus is	foci are
fossa is	fossae are
decubitus *ulcer* is	decubitus *ulcers* are

(NOTE: Decubitus is *not* a noun and has no plural form.)

TEMPERATURE VERSUS FEVER

If a dictator says "Patient has some headache but no temperature," remember we *always* have a temperature, it just may not be elevated. Correctly transcribed, the phrase should read either, "Patient has some headache but no elevated temperature" or "Patient has some headache but no fever."

A TONGUE TWISTER

The changes listed below are found in patients with chronic muscle spasm. The difference between chronic spasm and newly acquired spasm can be palpated and may be described as either

tense, tender tissue texture changes

-or-

tender tissue texture changes

DERMATOLOGY TERMS

Hair cycles or phases include (1) anagen, (2) catagen, and (3) telogen. Examples include anagen effluvium, a loss of hair after chemotherapy, and telogen effluvium, a loss of hair due to the trauma of surgery, high fever, stress, etc.

pyknotic nuclei = a thickening of the nuclei

arrectores pilorum = muscles in the connective tissue of the upper dermis, attached to the hair follicles below the sebaceous glands

delling = the formation of a slight blister or dimpling

PULMONARY TERMS

I:E ratio (dictated "I to E")

The ratio of inspiratory to expiratory time.

E → A (dictated "E to A")

When the patient's saying E, E, E comes out as A, A, A upon auscultation of the lung. This shows consolidation of the lung.

GYNECOLOGY TERMS

gravida 6, **para 4-0-2-3**, in case you wonder, refers to

6 pregnancies resulting in

4 full-term deliveries with

0 premature births and

2 abortions or miscarriages and

3 living children

If a GYN dictation does not "add up," question the originator of the dictation or check the chart.

CARDIOLOGY TERMS

Murmur grades are written in arabic numerals.

Example: A 2-3/6 systolic ejection murmur was heard at the left sternal border.

NOTE: It is unlikely that a report would be sent back if roman numerals are used; they aren't "wrong, wrong," but arabic numerals have been recommended for the past few years.

CLINICAL LABORATORY TERMS

PT/PTT refers to two separate tests used to track anticoagulation. The PT (prothrombin time or pro time) can be used to keep track of Coumadin levels (a blood thinner). The PTT (partial thromboplastin time) can be used to keep track of heparin levels (also a blood thinner). PT/PTT results can be abnormal with blood abnormalities, in liver disease, in hemophilia, etc. (Remember, pro time is always two words.)

RACE

When transcribing race, Caucasian and African-American are properly capitalized; however, white and black are properly lowercase.

>Examples:
>
>This 45-year-old black female ...
>
>This 72-year-old white male ...
>
>A 15-month-old Caucasian girl ...
>
>A 25-year-old black Cuban male ...
>
>-OR-
>
>This black male patient is 15 years old.
>
>My Anglo gardener is 74 years old.
>
>An African-American girl 9 months old ...
>
>His boy, a Native American, is 7 years old.

AGE

In age references, remember:

- Neonates/newborns are people from birth to 1 month of age.
- Infants are people 1 month to 24 months of age.
- Children are people 2 years to 13 years of age, also boys or girls.
- Adolescents are people 13 to 17 years of age, also teenagers, boys, or girls.
- Adults are people 18 years of age or older, also men or women.

ZERO SAFETY

Preceding zeros with decimals: These are important safety factors in transcription. In either typewritten or handwritten records, a decimal point on the line is hard to see, is easily missed, and incorrect dosing can result. The preceding zero is essential in transcription. For example:

Dictated "Xylocaine point 1 percent," should be transcribed *Xylocaine 0.1%*.

A drug dosage dictated as .25 should be transcribed 0.25.

NOTE: This pertains only to zeros **in front of** decimals (preceding zeros), and not to those behind the decimal.

ROMAN NUMERALS

When roman numerals are used in dictating the digits, here is what they mean:

>I digitus primus manus = digit I (thumb)
>
>II digitus secundus manus = digit II (index finger)
>
>III digitus tertius manus = digit III (long finger)
>
>IV digitus quartus manus = digit IV (ring finger)
>
>V digitus quintus manus = digit V (little finger)

Roman numerals used with proper names take no comma *before* the numeral.

>Example:
>
>Magnus Flaws III, CPA
>
>Gerald B. Hensley II, M.D.

TIME

When transcribing time followed by a.m. or p.m., use no zeros and no colon when the full hour is given.

>Example:
>
>Take the medication at 8 a.m., noon, and 4 p.m.; however, take a meal at 7:30 a.m., 11:30 a.m., and 3:30 p.m.

Whenever 12 o'clock is specified as *time*, simply use noon or midnight. No numerals are necessary.

A 50-pack-year smoking history = smoking a pack a day for 50 years. The pack-year is the result of the *packs per day multiplied by the number of years of smoking.*

CMTips™ are compiled by Patricia A. Ireland, CMT; references include the *AMA Manual of Style*, ed 8; *Dorland's Illustrated Medical Dictionary*, ed. 28; *Stedman's Medical Dictionary*, ed. 26; *The Gregg Reference Manual*, ed. 7; *Pyle's Current Medical Terminology*, ed 6.

TRANSCRIPTION USING THE STUDENT DISK

A 3.5" software disk is included at the back of this text-workbook. It is designed to interact with two common word processing programs; Corel® WordPerfect® (versions 6.1 through 8) and Microsoft® Word (versions 6.0 or newer). You will need to have one of these word processing programs pre-installed on your computer before you can access all the information on the disk. Before you begin working, please refer to the Help file on the disk.

The software disk is designed to assist you in your transcription of the patient cases and reports described in the text-workbook and contained on the audiotapes. It includes templates for each of the eight reports used in *Hillcrest Medical Center,* as well as several "matching" exercises, "wordfind" puzzles, and proofreading exercises. The disk contains a file for each of the following reports: History & Physical, Request for Consultation, Radiology Report, Operative Report, Pathology Report, Discharge Summary, Death Summary, and Autopsy Report. You will also see files for each of the two outpatient reports you will need to complete the *Quali-Care Clinic,* Hillcrest Medical Center's satellite ambulatory care center. These are the HPIP (history, physical, impression, plan) report and the SOAP (subjective, objective, assessment, plan) report. Tips for formatting your reports are located under "Report Formatting Guidelines" within this section.

Because of the number of files you will be creating as you work through *Hillcrest Medical Center* and *Quali-Care Clinic,* you will need additional "work" disks on which to save your transcribed reports. We suggest that once you install the program onto your computer's hard drive, you save your reports by cases onto "work" disks. If necessary, refer to your computer user's manual for disk formatting and copying instructions.

After you have transcribed your report to disk, you will want to save the file with an identifiable name. For example, some sample file names could be: H&P-C1 (H&P for "history and physical," C1 for "case 1"), DIS-C10 (DIS for "discharge summary," C10 for "case 10") and RAD3C10 (RAD for "radiology report," 3 for "radiology report number 3," C10 for "case 10"). Again, refer to your word processing software user's manual if you have questions about saving and naming files.

After keying your medical reports, you will want to proofread and spell-check your reports for accuracy, just as you will need to carefully check your work after you enter the job market.

Report Formatting Guidelines

The following guidelines will help you format your report documents. Many of these guidelines are displayed on the Model Report Forms section of this text-workbook.

1. Use two spaces after periods at the end of a sentence.

2. Use two spaces after colons within the body of a report. Do not include spaces after dictator initials in the sign-off block.

3. Double space between all paragraphs.

4. Display all dates on report headings and in the sign-off block as MM/DD/YYYY (not M/D/YYYY or M/DD/Y). Dates appearing within the body of a report should be transcribed as dictated (e.g., May 14).

5. Use left justification on reports. (An embedded code has been added to the template diskette that will format reports with left justification.)

6. Use no hyphenation at the end of lines in reports.

7. Use a one-inch margin on sides, top, and bottom of report pages.

8. Double space between the last line on a page and the "(Continued)" notation.

9. All page breaks should take place between paragraphs or in the middle of a paragraph with at least two lines on the bottom of one page and two lines at the top of the next page. Avoid "widows" and "orphans" (single lines of text that appear at the bottom or top of a page, separated from the rest of the paragraph).

10. Do not include the signature block alone on a page. Include at least two lines of text on the top of the page containing the signature block.

11. Quadruple space (4 hard returns) between the ending paragraph of a report and the signature rule (or line).

12. Position the signature rule at a four inch indent on the tab ruler using the indent command (appears as POS 5" on position indicator). The signature rule for Hillcrest should consist of 25 underscore lines.

13. Do not include extra spaces between the physician's name and the signature rule. The physician's name should be positioned at a four inch indent to align with the signature rule.

14. Use a double space between the physician's name and the sign-off block at the end of a report.

15. Use a double space between the transcribed date and copy line (if applicable) at the end of a report.

16. Single space all subsequent page headers (report title in all caps, patient name, hospital number, and page number). Use a quadruple space to the paragraph below.

17. Use a double space above and below sign-off blocks occurring between two parts of a report.

18. For subheadings containing enumerated text within the body of a report, format the subhead in all caps with a colon. Use the indent command to position the first enumerated item. Also, use the indent command following the number and period so that runover text aligns with text above.

19. Use all caps and colons for brief introducers within the body of a report (e.g., "HEENT: Normocephalic" used in History and Physical report). Use all caps without a colon for introducers used in a complete sentence (e.g., "SKIN is warm and dry to the touch" used in History and Physical report).

20. Center the cap main headings (FINAL ANATOMIC DIAGNOSIS, GROSS AUTOPSY EXAMINATION, MICROSCOPIC DESCRIPTION) on an Autopsy report.

Common WordPerfect and Word Commands

The following two charts list common commands used in Corel® WordPerfect® and Microsoft® Word, respectively. These commands are displayed to assist you in transcribing medical documents.

COREL WORDPERFECT KEYBOARD COMMANDS

Action	Windows Commands
Block	F8; drag with mouse
Bold	Ctrl-B
Bottom of Document	Ctrl-End
Cancel	Esc
Center	Shift-F7
Close	Ctrl-F4
Column (Left/Right)	Alt-Left Arrow/Right Arrow
Copy	Ctrl-Ins; Ctrl-C
Cut	Shift-Del; Ctrl-X
Decimal Tab	Alt-Shift-F7

Action	**Windows Commands**
Delete End of Line	Ctrl-Del
Double Indent	Ctrl-Shift-F7
End Field	Alt-Enter
Exit	Alt-F4
Flush Right	Alt-F7
Font	F9; Ctrl-F (6.1)
Footnote	Alt-I; F
Go to	Ctrl-G
Hard Page	Ctrl-Enter
Help	F1
Indent	F7
Italics	Ctrl-I
Macro Play	Alt-F10
Macro Record	Ctrl-F10
Macro Stop	Ctrl-Shift-F10 (5.1); Ctrl-F10
Merge	Shift-F9
Merge/Sort	Alt-F9
Next Document	Alt-W; select document
Open	Ctrl-O
Page Down	Alt-PgDn
Page Up	Alt-PgUp
Paste	Shift-Ins; Ctrl-V
Print	F5; Ctrl-P
Print Preview	Shift-F5 (5.1)
Replace	Ctrl-F2
Reveal Codes	Alt-F3
Ruler	Alt-Shift-F3

Action	Windows Commands
Save	Shift-F3; Ctrl-S
Save As	F3
Screen Down	Pg Dn
Search	F2
Screen Up	Pg Up
Search Next	Shift-F2
Search Previous	Alt-F2
Select	F8; drag with mouse
Select Paragraph	Quadruple click
Select Sentence	Triple click
Speller	Ctrl-F1
Styles	Alt-F8
Thesaurus	Alt-F1
Top of Document	Ctrl-Home
Undelete	Alt-Shift-Bksp (5.1); Ctrl-Shift-Z
Underline	Ctrl-U
Undo	Alt-Bksp (5.1); Ctrl-Z

MICROSOFT WORD KEYBOARD COMMANDS

Action	Keystrokes	Action	Keystrokes
Apply bold	Ctrl+B	Increase font size	Ctrl+Shift+>
Apply italic formatting	Ctrl+I	Increase font size by 1 point	Ctrl+]
Apply underline	Ctrl+U	Indent	Ctrl+M
Cancel	Esc	Justify	Ctrl+J
Center	Ctrl+E	Left align	Ctrl+L
Change case of letters	Shift+F3	Open	Ctrl+O
Change font	Ctrl+Shift+F	Print	Ctrl+P
Change font size	Ctrl+Shift+P	Quit Word	Alt+F4
Close	Ctrl+W	Redo or repeat an action	Ctrl+Y
Copy	Ctrl+C	Reduce hanging indent	Ctrl+Shift+T
Create hanging indent	Ctrl+T	Remove indent from the left	Ctrl+Shift+M
Create new document	Ctrl+N	Remove paragraph formatting	Ctrl+Q
Decrease font size	Ctrl+Shift+<	Right align	Ctrl+R
Decrease font size by 1 point	Ctrl+[	Save	Ctrl+S
Double-space lines	Ctrl+2	Single-space lines	Ctrl+1
Format letters as all capitals	Ctrl+Shift+A	Undo	Ctrl+Z

Instructors may choose to have students transcribe reports on a typewriter using a copy of the blank forms included at the back of the text-workbook (see also information under "Blank Medical Forms"). Or, instructors may instruct students with access to WordPerfect to use the forms provided on the template diskette. The template includes each of the eight report forms needed to complete *Hillcrest Medical Center*.

The template diskette will allow students to spell-check their reports using a medical dictionary customized for *Hillcrest Medical Center*. The dictionary includes all medical words used in the cases. A macro has been developed that instructs WordPerfect to consult the supplemental dictionary located on the template diskette. Instructions for using this macro are included in this text-workbook under "Transcription Using WordPerfect."

Additionally, the template diskette contains macros that allow you to tabulate word counts and line counts for each report. Instructors may wish to have students accumulate word counts or line counts per case to practice submitting invoices for payment as they may when they enter the job market. The word counting and line counting features are included to simulate "real world" transcription practices.

Note: The macros on the template have been developed to work with WordPerfect 5.1 and above. The spell-check macros assume that the main dictionary for WordPerfect is located in the default location specified during standard installation. If the main dictionary is located in a different directory, the macro will not recognize where to find the dictionary and the macro may be inoperable. Students should talk to their instructor if they need additional assistance.

VOICE RECOGNITION TECHNOLOGY

For more than 20 years, voice (or speech) recognition technology has been studied, researched, tested, and found wanting. But those who have been working on it swear it is just a matter of time before it is perfected. What this will mean is that dictation will be able to be spoken into a machine, understood, and transcribed by same. This technology is designed to save time, reduce transcription costs, accelerate billing and collection, and offer more flexibility and accuracy to the originator of the dictation.

Most professionals in medical transcription have felt that this technology is being designed to *replace* them. However, the transcriptionist will still be needed and will play an important role as medical language specialist and medical/technical editor. The important things for MT students to recognize is that they are studying to enter an important profession, one that is suffering from a lack of well-trained practitioners. Their services will continue to be required, and students are encouraged to think of themselves as medical/technical editors in training.

The future will always hold changes. Voice recognition technology plus the medical language specialist will potentially be able to help those in healthcare by providing accurate patient records in a timely fashion.

Understanding Medical Terminology

Some of the most common prefixes, combining forms, and suffixes used in medical terminology are listed with their definitions. Students who have completed a medical terminology course prior to beginning Hillcrest will find this section to be a comprehensive review.

Understanding
Medical Terminology

Medical terminology appears to be complicated until one learns the principles of basic word structure. Medical terminology consists of the following components:

- prefix, word beginning
- suffix, word ending
- root word, the foundation of a word
- combining vowel, a vowel (usually o) connecting a root word to a suffix or a root word to another root word
- combining form, the combination of a root word and a combining vowel.

The combining vowel aids in pronunciation.

PRINCIPLES

1. Generally speaking, begin reading a medical word from the suffix to the root word and/or prefix.

   Example: hemi/   gloss/   ectomy

   half   tongue   removal

   (prefix)   (root)   (suffix)

   Definition: removal of half (one side of) the tongue

2. Drop the combining vowel before a suffix beginning with a vowel.

   Example: gastr/   itis   NOT gastr/   o/   itis

   stomach   inflammation

   (root)   (suffix)

   Definition: inflammation of the stomach

3. Retain the combining vowel before a suffix beginning with a consonant.

   Example: gastr/   o/   megaly   NOT gastr/   megaly

   enlargement

   (suffix)

   Definition: enlargement of the stomach

4. Retain the combining vowel between two root words even if the second root word begins with a vowel.

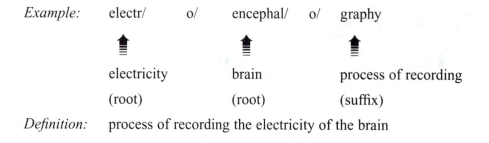

Example: electr/   o/   encephal/   o/   graphy

electricity   brain   process of recording
(root)   (root)   (suffix)

Definition: process of recording the electricity of the brain

Listed below are some commonly used prefixes, combining forms, and suffixes.

Prefixes/Pronunciation	Meaning	Example
A		
a- (ā, ă)	not, without	apnea—not breathing
ab- (ăb)	away from	aberrant—deviating from the normal
ad- (ăd)	to, toward	adhere—to cling together
ambi- (ăm´ bĭ)	on both sides	ambilateral—affecting both sides
an- (ăn)	not, without	anoxia—without oxygen
ante- (ăn´ tē)	before	antefebrile—before the onset of fever
anti- (ăn´ tī, an´ tĭ)	against	antiemetic—an agent that prevents nausea
auto- (aw´ tō)	self	autohypnotic—pertaining to self-induced hypnotism
B		
bi- (bī)	two	biarticular—pertaining to two joints
brady- (brăd´ ē, brād´ ē)	slow	bradycardia—slowness of the heartbeat
C		
cata- (kăt´ ah)	down	cataphoria—a permanent downward turning of the visual axes of the eyes
co- (kō)	with, together	cohesive—uniting together
con- (kŏn)	with, together	conexus—a connecting structure
contra- (kŏn´ trah)	against, opposite	contraceptive—an agent that prevents conception
D		
de- (dē)	lack of	dehydrate—to remove water from
di- (dī)	two, twice	diplopia—double vision
dia- (dī´ ah)	complete, through	dialysis—complete separation
dis- (dĭs)	reversal, separation	disacidify—to remove an acid from
dys- (dĭs)	bad, painful, difficult	dysmenorrhea—painful menstrual flow

E

ecto- (ĕkˊtō)	out, outside	ectopic—out of normal position
en- (ĕn)	in, within	encephalic—within the skull
endo- (ĕnˊdō)	within	endocrine—pertaining to secretions within
epi- (ĕpˊĭ)	above, upon	epibulbar—upon the eyeball
eu- (ū)	good, well, easily	eupepsia—good digestion
ex- (ĕks)	out, outside	excision—removal
exo- (ĕkˊsō)	outside, outward	exocardial—situated outside the heart

H

hemi- (hĕmˊē)	half	hemiglossitis—inflammation of one half of the tongue
hyper- (hīˊpĕr)	above, excessive	hyperactivity—excessive activity
hypo- (hīˊpō)	deficient, below	hypotension—abnormally low blood pressure

I

in (ĭn)	not	incurable—not able to be cured
infra- (ĭnˊfrah)	below, inferior	infrasternal—below the sternum (breast bone)
inter- (ĭnˊtĕr)	between	intercostal—between the ribs
intra- (ĭnˊtrah)	within	intracutaneous—within the skin

M

macro- (măkˊrō)	large	macrocyte—an abnormally large erythrocyte (red blood cell)
mal- (măl)	bad	malnutrition—any disorder of nutrition
meso- (mĕzˊō)	middle	mesonasal—situated in the middle of the nose
meta- (mĕtˊah)	beyond, change	metamorphosis—change of shape
micro- (mīˊkrō)	small	microcyst—a very small cyst

N

neo- (nēˊō)	new	neonate—a newborn infant

P

pan- (păn)	all	panhysterectomy—total hysterectomy
para- (părˊah)	near, beside	paraesophageal—near the esophagus
per- (pĕr)	through	percutaneous—performed through the skin

peri- (pĕr´ē)	around, surrounding	perihepatic—occurring around the liver
poly- (pŏl´ē)	many	polyneuritis—inflammation of many nerves
post- (pōst)	after, behind	postoperative—after a surgical procedure
pre- (prē)	before, in front of	preprandial—before meals
pro- (prō)	before	prognosis—a forecast as to the probable outcome of a disease

R

| re- (rē) | back, again | reabsorb—to absorb again |
| retro- (rĕt´rō) | behind, backward | retronasal—behind the nose |

S

semi- (sĕm´ē)	one half, partly	semiprone—partly prone (lying face downward)
sub- (sŭb)	under, below	subabdominal—situated below the abdomen
supra- (soo´prah)	above, over	suprarenal—situated above a kidney
sym- (sĭm)	together, with	sympodia—fusion of the lower extremities
syn- (sĭn)	together, with	syndrome—a set of symptoms that occur together

T

| tachy- (tăk´ē) | fast, rapid | tachycardia—excessive rapidity in the action of the heart |
| trans- (trăns) | across, through | transepidermal—occurring through or across the epidermis (top layer of skin) |

U

| ultra- (ŭl´trah) | beyond, excess | ultrastructure—the structure beyond the resolution power of the light microscope |

COMBINING FORMS

A

aden/o (ăd´ ĕn-ō)	gland	adenodynia—pain in a gland
angi/o (ăn´ jē-ō)	vessel	angiectomy—surgical excision of a vessel
arteri/o (ăr-tē´ rē-ō)	artery	arterioplasty—surgical repair of an artery
arthr/o (ăr´ thrō)	joint	arthrotomy—surgical incision of a joint

B

blephar/o (blĕf´ ăr-ō)	eyelid	blepharoplegia—paralysis of an eyelid
brachi/o (brā´ kē-ō)	arm	brachiocephalic—pertaining to the arm and head
bucc/o (bŭk´ ō)	cheek	buccolingual—pertaining to the cheek and tongue
burs/o (bĕr´ sō)	bursa (fluid-filled sac)	bursopathy—any disease of a bursa

C

carcin/o (kăr´ sĭn-ō)	carcinoma	carcinolysis—destruction of carcinoma cells
cardi/o (kăr´ dēō)	heart	cardiogenic—originating in the heart
cephal/o (sĕf´ ah-lō)	head	cephaledema—edema of the head
cerebr/o (sĕr´ ĕ-brō)	brain, cerebrum	cerebrospinal—pertaining to the brain and spinal cord
cervic/o (sĕr´ vĭ-kō)	neck	cervicoplasty—plastic surgery of the neck
coccyg/o (kŏk´ sē-gō)	tailbone, coccyx	coccygodynia—pain in the coccyx
cost/o (kŏs´ tō)	ribs	costoclavicular—pertaining to the ribs and clavicle (collar bone)
crani/o (krā´ nē-ō)	skull	craniopathy—any disease of the skull
cutane/o (kūt-tā´ nē-ō)	skin	subcutaneous—beneath the skin
cyst/o (sĭs´ tō)	urinary bladder	cystogram—an x-ray of the urinary bladder

D

dactyl/o (dăk´ tĭl-ō)	finger or toe	dactylospasm—spasm of a finger or toe
dent/i (dĕn´ tē)	tooth	dentibuccal—pertaining to the teeth and cheek
dips/o (dĭp´ sō)	thirst	dipsosis—morbid thirst
dors/o (dŏr´ sō)	back of the body	dorsolateral—pertaining to the back and side

E

electr/o (ē-lĕk´ trō)	electricity	electrotome—a surgical cutting instrument powered by electricity
encephal/o (ĕn-sĕf´ ah-lō)	brain	encephalomyelitis—inflammation of the brain and spinal cord
enter/o (ĕn´ tĕr-ō)	intestine	enterorrhaphy—repair or suture of the intestine
esophag/o (ĕ-sŏf´ ă-gō)	esophagus	esophagomalacia—softening of the walls of the esophagus

F

fasci/o (făsh´ ē-ō)	fascia (fibrous tissue)	fasciitis—inflammation of fascia
femor/o (fĕm´ ō-rō)	femur (thigh bone)	femoroiliac—pertaining to the femur and ilium (hip bone)
fibul/o (fĭb´ ū-lō)	fibula (the smaller of the two lower leg bones)	fibulocalcaneal—pertaining to the fibula and calcaneus (heel bone)

G

gastr/o (găs´ trō)	stomach	gastrostenosis—contraction or shrinkage of the stomach
gingiv/o (jĭn´ jĭ-vō)	gums	gingivolabial—pertaining to the gums and lips
gloss/o (glŏs´ ō)	tongue	glossopharyngeal—pertaining to the tongue and pharynx (throat)
gynec/o (gī´ nĕ-kō)	woman, female	gynecology—that branch of medicine that treats diseases of the female genital tract

H

hemat/o (hēm´ ah-tō)	blood	hematuria—blood in the urine
hepat/o (hĕp´ ah-tō)	liver	hepatologist—a specialist in the study of the liver
hist/o (hĭs´ tō)	tissue	histolysis—destruction of tissue
hypn/o (hĭp´ nō)	sleep	hypnogenic—inducing sleep
hyster/o (hĭs´ tĕr-ō)	uterus, womb	hysterosalpingectomy—excision of the uterus and uterine (fallopian) tubes

I

idi/o (ĭd´ ē-ō)	individual, self	idiopathic—self-originated condition of unknown causation

ile/o (ĭl´ ē-ō)	ileum (portion of the small intestine)	ileocecal—pertaining to the ileum and cecum
ili/o (ĭl´ ē-ō)	ilium (expansive superior portion of the hip bone)	iliocostal—pertaining to the ilium and ribs

J

jejun/o (jě-joo´ nō)	jejunum (portion of the small intestine)	jejunectomy—excision of the jejunum

K

kerat/o (kěr´ ah-tō)	cornea	keratomycosis—fungal infection of the cornea
kinesi/o (kĭ-nē´ sē-ō)	movement	kinesiotherapy—treatment of disease by movements or exercise

L

labi/o (lā´ bē-ō)	lip	labiolingual—pertaining to the lips and tongue
laryng/o (lah-rĭng´ ō)	larynx (voice box)	laryngoparalysis—paralysis of the larynx
later/o (lăt´ ěr-ō)	side	lateroversion—a turning to one side
lip/o (lĭp´ ō)	fat, lipid	lipiduria—lipids in the urine
lith/o (lĭth´ ō)	stone, calculus	lithogenous—producing or causing the formation of calculi

M

mamm/o (măm´ ō)	breast	mammoplasty—plastic reconstruction of the breast
mast/o (măs´ tō)	breast	mastography—the making of an x-ray of the breast
my/o (mī´ ō)	muscle	myobradia—slow, sluggish reaction of muscle to electric stimulation
myel/o (mī´ ě-lō)	spinal cord, bone marrow	myelopoiesis—formation of bone marrow

N

nas/o (nā´ zō)	nose	nasopalatine—pertaining to the nose and palate (roof of the mouth)
nephr/o (něf´ rō)	kidney	nephrorrhagia—hemorrhage from a kidney
neur/o (nū´ rō)	nerve	neuroallergy—allergy in nervous tissue
noct/i (nŏk´ tē)	night	nocturia—excessive urination at night

O

onc/o (ŏng´ kō)	mass, tumor	oncogenesis—the production or causation of tumors
oo/o (ō´ ō-ō)	egg, ovum	oocyte—an immature egg
oophor/o (ō-ŏf´ ō-rō)	ovary	oophorohysterectomy—excision of the ovaries and uterus
ophthalm/o (ŏf-thăl´ mō)	eye	ophthalmodynia—pain in the eye
orchi/o (ŏr´ kē-ō)	testis, testicle	orchitis—inflammation of the testicle
or/o (ō´ rō)	mouth	oral—pertaining to the mouth
oste/o (ŏs´ tē-ō)	bone	osteodystrophy—abnormal, defective bone formation
ot/o (ō´ tō)	ear	otorrhea—a discharge from the ear
ox/o (ŏk´ sō)	oxygen	anoxia—absence of oxygen

P

path/o (păth´ ō)	disease	pathoanatomic—pertaining to the anatomy of diseased tissue
poster/o (pŏs´ tĕr-ō)	back (of the body)	posterolateral—behind and to one side
pseud/o (sū´ dō)	false	pseudocyesis—false pregnancy
psych/o (sī´ kō)	mind	psychogenesis—mental development
py/o (pī´ ō)	pus	pyosalpinx—pus in the uterine tube

R

radi/o (rā´ dē-ō)	rays, x-rays	radioimmunity—diminished sensitivity to radiation
ren/o (rē´ nō)	kidney	renal—pertaining to the kidney
retin/o (rĕt´ ĭ-nō)	retina	retinomalacia—softening of the retina
rhin/o (rī´ nō)	nose	rhinotomy—incision of the nose
roentgen/o (rĕnt´ gĕn-ō)	x-rays	roentgenotherapy—treatment with roentgen rays

S

sacr/o (sā´ krō)	sacrum	sacrodynia—pain in the sacral region
salping/o (săl-pĭng´ gō)	uterine tubes	salpingo-oophorectomy—excision of a uterine tube and an ovary
secti/o (sĕk´ shē-ō)	to cut	section—a cut surface
sphygm/o (sfĭg´ mō)	pulse	sphygmometer—an instrument for measuring the pulse
stomat/o (stō´ mah-tō)	mouth	stomatomycosis—fungal disease of the mouth

T

thorac/o (thō´ rah-kō)	chest	thoracoscopy—examination of the pleural cavity with an endoscope
tibi/o (tĭb´ ē-ō)	tibia, shin bone (the larger of the two lower leg bones)	tibialgia—painful shin bone
top/o (tŏp´ ō)	place, position, location	ectopic—located away from normal position
tox/o (tŏk´ sō)	poison	toxicity—the quality of being poisonous
trache/o (trā´ kē-ō)	trachea (windpipe)	tracheolaryngotomy—incision of the larynx (voice box) and trachea

U

ur/o (ū´ rō)	urine, urinary tract	urolith—a calculus (stone) in the urine
uter/o (ū´ tĕr-ō)	uterus	uteroplacental—pertaining to the placenta and uterus

V

vagin/o (văj´ ĭ-nō)	vagina	vaginovesical—pertaining to the vagina and urinary bladder
vas/o (văs´ ō)	vessel, duct	vasomotion—change in the caliber of a (blood) vessel
ven/o (vē´ nō)	vein	veno-occlusive—pertaining to obstruction of the veins
viscer/o (vĭs´ ĕr-ō)	internal organs	viscerad—toward the viscera

X

xanth/o (zăn´ thō)	yellow	xanthemia—presence of yellow coloring matter in the blood
xer/o (zēr´ rō)	dry	xerosis—abnormal dryness

Z

zyg/o (zī´ gō)	yoked, joined	zygal—shaped like a yoke

SUFFIXES

A

-ac (ăk)	pertaining to	cardiac—pertaining to the heart
-al (ăl)	pertaining to	postnatal—pertaining to after a birth
-algia (ăl´ jē-ah)	pain	otalgia—pain in the ear
-asthenia (ăs-thē´ nē-ah)	lack of strength	myasthenia—deficient muscular power

C

-cele (sēl)	hernia	cystocele—hernial protrusion of the urinary bladder through the vaginal wall
-centesis (sĕn-tē´ sĭs)	surgical puncture to remove fluid	amniocentesis—surgical puncture to remove fluid from the amnion
-cidal (sī´ dăl)	killing	bactericidal—destructive to bacteria
-clysis (klī´ sĭs)	irrigation, washing	enteroclysis—the injection of a medicinal liquid into the bowel
-coccus (kōk´ ŭs)	bacterial cell	staphylococcus—microorganism that causes localized suppurative infections
-cyte (sīt)	cell	leukocyte—white blood cell

D

-desis (dē´ sĭs)	binding	arthrodesis—surgical fixation of a joint

E

-ectasis (ĕk´ tah-sĭs)	stretching, dilation	angiectasis—lengthening of a blood vessel
-ectomy (ĕk´ tō-mē)	removal	appendectomy—removal of the vermiform appendix
-emesis (ĕm´ ě-sĭs)	vomiting	hyperemesis—excessive vomiting
-emia (ē´ mē-ah)	blood condition	septicemia—blood poisoning

G

-genesis (jĕn´ ě-sĭs)	producing, originating	pathogenesis—the development of disease or a morbid condition
-gram (grăm)	record	myelogram—an x-ray of the spinal cord
-graph (grăf)	instrument for recording	gastrograph—an instrument for recording the motions of the stomach
-graphy (grăf´ ē)	process of recording	myelography—the making of an x-ray of the spinal cord after injection of a contrast medium (dye) into the subarachnoid space

I

-ia (ē´ ah)	condition, process	dyspepsia—condition of bad digestion
-ic (ĭk)	pertaining to	thoracic—pertaining to the chest
-ist (ĭst)	specialist	nephrologist—a specialist in the study of the kidney
-itis (ī´ tĭs)	inflammation	osteitis—inflammation of a bone

L

-logy (lō´ jē)	study of	ophthalmology—study of the eye
-lysis (lī´ sĭs)	separation, destruction	splenolysis—destruction of splenic tissue

M

-malacia (mah-lā´ shē-ăh)	softening	osteomalacia—softening of bone
-megaly (mĕg´ ah-lē)	enlargement	acromegaly—enlargement of extremities

O

-odynia (ō-dĭn´ ē-ah)	pain	gastrodynia—pain in the stomach
-ole (ōl)	little, small	arteriole—a minute arterial branch
-oma (ō´ mah)	tumor	carcinoma—a malignant new growth
-opia (ō´ pē-ah)	vision	amblyopia—dimming of vision
-orrhaphy (ŏr´ ah-fē)	suture	herniorrhaphy—suture of a hernia
-orrhea (ō´ rē-ah)	flow, discharge	menorrhea—discharge of the menses
-osis (ō´ sĭs)	abnormal condition	arthropyosis—abnormal condition of pus in a joint cavity
-osmia (ŏz´ mē-ah)	smell	anosmia—absence of the sense of smell
-ostomy (ŏs´tō-mē)	new opening	colostomy—surgical creation of a new opening in the colon

P

-pepsia (pĕp´ sē-ah)	digestion	dyspepsia—bad digestion
-phagia (fā´ jē-ah)	eating, swallowing	polyphagia—excessive eating
-phobia (fō´ bē-ah)	fear	hydrophobia—fear of water
-plasia (plā´ zē-ah)	formation, development	chondroplasia—the formation of cartilage
-plasty (plăs´ tē)	surgical repair	rhinoplasty—surgical repair of the nose
-plegia (plē´ jē-ah)	paralysis	hemiplegia—paralysis of one side of the body
-pnea (nē´ ah)	breathing	dyspnea—difficult breathing
-ptosis (tō´ sĭs)	drooping, prolapse	blepharoptosis—drooping of the eyelid
-ptysis (tĭ´ sĭs)	spitting	hemoptysis—spitting blood

S

-sclerosis (sklē-rō´ sĭs)	hardening	arteriosclerosis—hardening of the arteries
-scope (skōp)	instrument for visual examination	cystoscope—an instrument for visual examination of the urinary bladder
-stasis (stā´ sĭs)	control, stop	hemostasis—stopping the flow of blood
-stenosis (stĕn-ō´ sĭs)	narrowing, stricture	angiostenosis—narrowing of a vessel

T

-therapy (thĕr´ ah-pē)	treatment	thermotherapy—therapeutic use of heat
-tocia (tō´ sē-ah)	labor, birth	dystocia—abnormal labor
-tome (tōm)	instrument to cut	osteotome—an instrument to cut bone
-tomy (tō´ mē)	incision	tracheotomy—incision of the trachea
-trophy (trō´ fē)	nourishment, development	hypertrophy—excessive development

U

-ule (ūl)	little, small	venule—a small vein
-uria (ū´ rē-ah)	urination, urine	pyuria—pus in the urine

Case Studies

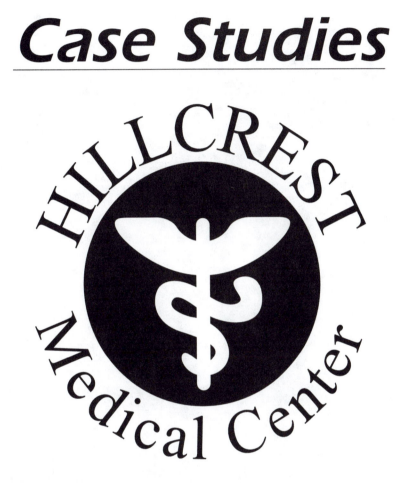

HILLCREST Medical Center

Case 1: The Reproductive System

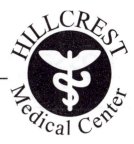

Patient Name

Julie Reynolds

Address

701 Dadeland Blvd.
Miami, FL 33133-5017

Situation

Julie Reynolds, a young woman who has had chronic gynecologic problems, has returned to her physician, an internist with a subspecialty in clinical gynecology. It was decided that surgery was required to correct her problem, so Ms. Reynolds was referred to a gynecologic surgeon. The tissue removed at surgery was sent to a pathologist for both macroscopic and microscopic examination and diagnosis. After an uncomplicated stay in the hospital, the patient was discharged by her internist for follow-up in the offices of both the internist and the surgeon.

Review Illustration 1-1, The Female Anatomy, on page 77 and Illustration 1-2, Suturing Techniques, on page 78.

Student Name: _____

Patient: Julie Reynolds

Sequence of Reports	Date Completed	Grade
History and Physical Examination	_____	_____
Operative Report	_____	_____
Pathology Report	_____	_____
Discharge Summary	_____	_____

Enter the date of completion for each report. When you have finished all reports, tear this sheet out, staple it to the front of the reports (in the order listed above), and give the completed reports to your instructor.

Glossary for Case 1
WORDS & PHONETIC PRONUNCIATIONS   DEFINITIONS

A

abortion (ab)		the premature expulsion from the uterus of the products of conception
adenomyosis	(ăd˝ĕ-nō-mī-ō´-sĭs)	a benign condition characterized by ingrowth of the endometrium into the uterine musculature
adhesion		the abnormal union of separate tissue surfaces by new fibrous tissue resulting from an inflammatory process
adnexa	(ăd-něk´sah)	appendages or adjunct parts
auscultation	(aws˝kŭl-tā´shŭn)	the act of listening for sounds within the body

B

Betadine®	(bā´tah-dīn)	trade name for preparations of povidone-iodine; used as a topical anti-infective agent
bisection		a division into two parts by cutting

C

cardinal ligament		part of a thickening of the visceral pelvic fascia beside the cervix and vagina, passing laterally to merge with the upper fascia of the pelvic diaphragm
cautery	(kaw´těr-ē)	the application of a caustic substance, a hot instrument, an electric current or other agent to destroy tissue
cervicitis	(sěr˝vĭ-sī´tĭs)	inflammation of the cervix uteri

chromic catgut	(krō´mĭk kăt´gŭt)	an absorbable sterile strand obtained from collagen derived from healthy mammals, sterilized and impregnated with chromium trioxide to prolong its tensile strength in tissues
cul-de-sac [Fr.]	(kŭl´dĕ-sahk´)	a blind pouch

D

dilation and curettage (D & C)	(dī-la´shŭn and kū´´rĕ-tahzh´)	dilation (stretching) of the cervix with various metal dilators and scraping of the lining of the uterus with an instrument called a curette
dorsolithotomy	(dŏr´´sō-lĭ-thŏt´ō-mē)	position of the body while lying on the back with legs lifted and separated; appropriate for GYN surgery

E

edema	(ĕ-dē´mah)	the presence of abnormally large amounts of fluid in the intercellular tissue spaces of the body
endometriosis	(ĕn-dō-mē´´trē-ō´sĭs)	a condition in which functioning endometrium is located ectopically, most often on the pelvic peritoneum and in the ovaries
endometrium	(ĕn-dō-mē´trē-ŭm)	the inner mucous membrane of the uterus
estrogen	(ĕs´trō-jĕn)	female sex hormone
ETOH		ethyl alcohol; ethanol; grain alcohol

F

fibrovascular stroma	(fī´´brō-văs´kū-lăr strō´mah)	a framework of tissue composed of fibers and blood vessels

G

genitourinary (GU)	(jĕn´´ĭ-tō-ū´rĭ-nār-ē)	pertaining to the genital and urinary organs
gravida [L.]	(grăv´ĭ-dah)	a pregnant woman

I

integumentary	(ĭn-tĕg-ū-mĕn´tăr-ē)	pertaining to or composed of skin
intraoperative	(ĭn´´trah-ŏp´ĕr-ă´´tiv)	occurring during the course of a surgical procedure
IV		intravenous

K

keratinous debris	(ke-răt´ĭ-nŭs dĕ-brē´)	"anatomic trash" consisting of insoluble material such as hair or nails or concretions that might be found within a cyst

L

labium majus [L.]	(lā´bē-ŭm mā´jŭs)	large pudendal lip (pl. labia majora)
laparoscopy	(lăp´´ah-rŏs´kō-pē)	examination of the interior of the abdomen by means of an instrument called a laparoscope
lysis	(lī´sĭs)	destruction; decomposition

M

Macrobid®	(măk´rō-bĭd)	trade name for nitrofurantoin; used in the prevention and treatment of urinary tract infections
metaplasia	(mĕt´´ah-plā´zē-ah)	the change in the type of adult cells in a tissue to a form that is not normal for that tissue
mucosa [L.]	(mū-kō´sah)	a mucous membrane
myometrium	(mī-ō-mē´trē-ŭm)	the smooth muscle coat of the uterus that forms the main mass of the organ

O

os [L.]	(ahs)	any orifice (opening or mouth) of the body, e.g., the cervical os; a general term (used with an adjective) to designate a specific type of bone structure, e.g., os calcis (heel bone)

P

pack-year		the equivalent of smoking one pack of cigarettes a day for one year
para [L.]	(păr´ah)	a woman who has given birth to viable young
pedicle	(pĕd´ĭ-k'l)	a footlike, stemlike, or narrow basal part or structure
percussion		the act of striking a part with short, sharp blows as an aid in diagnosing the condition of the underlying parts by the sound obtained
peritoneum	(pĕr´ĭ-tō-nē´ŭm)	the serous membrane lining the abdominal walls and investing the viscera
pharynx	(far´ĭnks)	throat
postoperative		occurring after a surgical procedure
prepped and draped		medical jargon meaning that the surgical field has been shaved, scrubbed, draped with sterile drapes, and otherwise prepared for the upcoming procedure. "Prepped" is short for "prepared."
prolapse	(prō-lăps´)	the falling down or sinking of a part or an organ
pursestring suture		a continuous circular inverting suture

R

reapproximate		to bring close together again

reperitonealized	(rē-pĕr˝ĭ-tō-nē´ăl-īzd)	having closed the peritoneum after a surgical procedure, suturing it closed
retractor		an instrument for maintaining operative exposure by separating the edges of a wound and holding back underlying organs and tissues
retroversion	(rĕt˝rō-vĕr´zhŭn)	the turning backward of the entire uterus in relation to the pelvic axis

S

salpingo-oophorectomy	(săl-pĭng˝gō-ō˝ŏf-ō-rĕk´tō-mē)	surgical removal of both a uterine tube and ovary
sebaceous	(sĕ-bā´shŭs)	secreting a greasy lubricating substance, sebum
serial	(sē´rē-ăl)	arranged in or forming a series
sinus rhythm		normal heart rhythm originating in the sinoatrial node
squamocolumnar junction	(skwā´mō-kōl˝ŭm-nĕr)	the junction between a stratified squamous epithelial surface and one lined by columnar epithelium
squamous	(skwā´mŭs)	scaly or platelike
stenosis	(stĕ-nō´sĭs)	narrowing or stricture of a duct or canal
supple		capable of being bent or folded without creases, cracks, or breaks; flexible

T

tenaculum	(tē-năk´ū-lŭm)	a hooklike instrument for seizing and holding tissues
tract	(trăkt)	a number of organs, arranged in series, subserving a common function
transfix		to pierce through and through

U

| utero-ovarian | (ū´´tĕr-ō-ō-vā´rē-ăn) | pertaining to the uterus and ovary |
| uterosacral | (ū´´tĕr-ō-sā´krăl) | pertaining to the uterus and the sacrum |

V

| varicosity | (văr´´ĭ-kŏs´i-tē) | a varicose condition |
| vulva | (vŭl´vah) | the region of the external genital organs of the female |

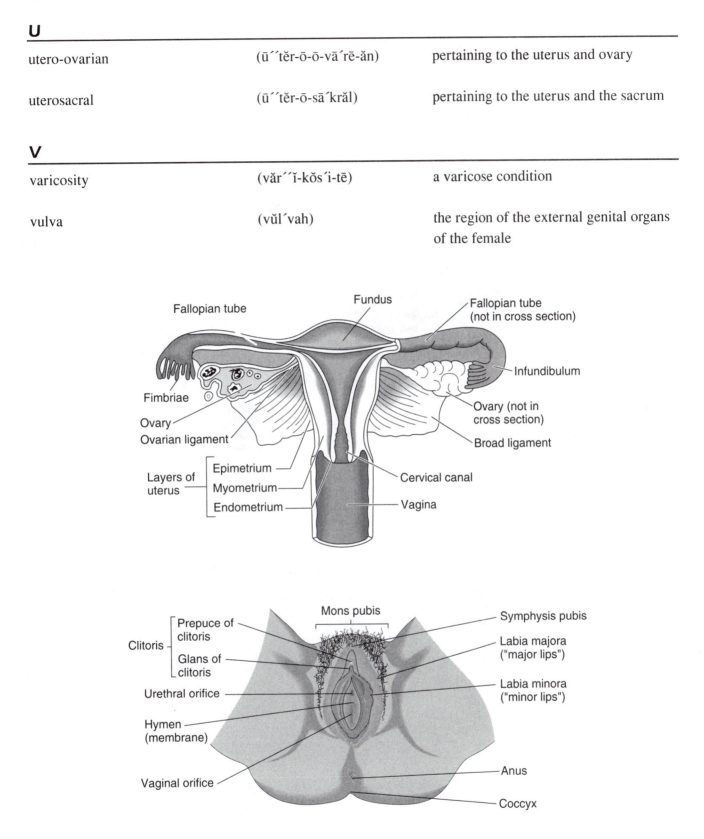

1-1. The female anatomy (A) anterior view. (B) external genitalia.

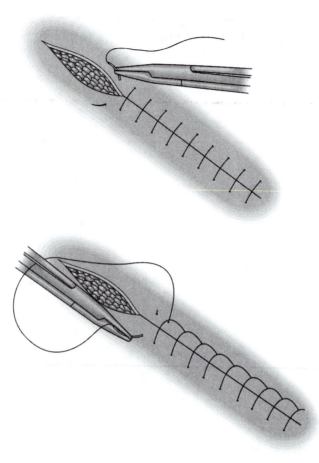

1-2. Suturing techniques.

Case 2: The Musculoskeletal System

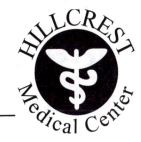

Patient Name

Emma Parker

Address

938 Shore Road
Ocean View, FL 33140-4989

Situation

This elderly woman fell and injured her hip. She was taken to Hillcrest emergency room where the ER physician ordered an x-ray. Her family physician was called who, in turn, requested an orthopedic surgeon to consult. Surgical intervention was decided on, and the patient was taken to the operating room. Radiology kept a close check on this patient throughout her hospital stay. She developed some cardiac problems postoperatively, and a cardiologist was requested to consult. Social workers at Hillcrest helped to get the patient placed in a nursing home at discharge, where she would be followed by her family physician, orthopedist, and cardiologist.

Review Illustration 2-1, The Skeleton, on page 86.

Student Name _____

Patient: Emma Parker

Sequence of Reports	Date Completed	Grade
History and Physical Examination	_____	_____
Radiology Report	_____	_____
Operative Report	_____	_____
Discharge Summary	_____	_____

Enter the date of completion for each report. When you have finished all reports, tear this sheet out, staple it to the front of the reports (in the order listed above), and give the completed reports to your instructor.

Glossary for Case 2
WORDS & PHONETIC PRONUNCIATIONS   DEFINITIONS

A

abduct	(ăb-dŭkt´)	to draw away from the median plane or (in the digits) from the axial line of a limb
Accu-Chek®	(ăk´ū-chĕk)	trade name for a blood sugar monitor
ADA		American Diabetes Association
Ancef®	(ăn´sĕf)	trade name for cefazolin, an antibiotic
anicteric	(ăn´´ĭk-tĕr´ĭk)	without icterus (jaundice; yellow appearance)
anteversion	(ăn´´tē-vĕr´zhŭn)	the forward tipping or tilting of an organ
antibiotic	(ăn´´tĭ-bī-ŏt´ĭk)	chemical substance produced by a microorganism which has the capacity to inhibit the growth of or to kill other microorganisms
AP		anteroposterior direction, from front to back
appendectomy		surgical removal of the vermiform appendix

B

bipolar	(bī-pō´lăr)	having two poles, ends, or extremes
buccal	(bŭk´ăl)	pertaining to or directed toward the cheek

C

C-arm images		results of portable x-ray unit used in the operating room
chronic		persisting over a long period of time

click		a brief sharp sound (heart sound)
copious	(kō´pē-ŭs)	yielding something abundantly
cortical	(kor´tĭ-kăl)	pertaining to a cortex (outer layer of an organ or other body structure)
CPK		creatinine phosphokinase (a lab test done on blood)

D

DePuy's sliding screw		orthopedic device used in femoral fracture repair
dissect	(dī-sĕkt´)	to cut apart or separate
dyspnea	(dĭsp´nē-ah)	difficult or labored breathing

E

electrocautery	(ē-lĕk´´trō-kaw´tĕr-ē)	the application of an electric current to destroy tissue
endotracheal	(ĕn´´dō-trā´kē-ăl)	within or through the trachea
EOMI		extraocular muscles *or* movements intact
external rotation		movement of an external appendage about its axis, e.g., moving either the leg or arm in a circle

F

fascia	(făsh´ē-ah)	a sheet or band of fibrous tissue that lies deep in the skin or forms an investment to receive muscles and various organs of the body
fascia lata	(făsh´ē-ah lah´tah)	the external investing fascia of the thigh
femoral	(fĕm´ŏr-ăl)	pertaining to the femur (thigh)
flex		to bend

fluoroscopy	(floo´´ŏr-ŏs´kō-pē)	examination by means of the fluoroscope (a device used for examining deep structures by means of roentgen rays)
funduscope	(fŭn´dŭs-skōp)	an instrument for examining the fundus (bottom or base) of the eye

G

gallop	(găl´ŏp)	a disordered rhythm of the heart

H

H&H		hemoglobin and hematocrit (blood tests)
hemostasis	(hē´´mō-stā´sĭs)	the arrest of bleeding, either by the physiological properties of vasoconstriction and coagulation or by surgical means
Hemovac drain		a closed suction drainage unit to evacuate blood and serum postoperatively

I

infarct	(ĭn´fărkt)	necrosis in a tissue due to local ischemia resulting from obstruction of circulation to the area
intact	(ĭn-tăkt´)	remaining uninjured, sound, or whole
intercostal	(ĭn´´tĕr-kŏs´tăl)	situated between the ribs
interrupted sutures		sutures (surgical stitches) that are placed separately and tied separately
intertrochanteric fracture	(ĭn´´tĕr-trō´´kăn-tĕr´ĭk)	a break within the trochanter (bones of the neck of the femur or thigh)
ischemia	(ĭs-kē´mē-ah)	deficiency of blood in a part, due to functional constriction or actual obstruction of a blood vessel

IVPB		intravenous piggyback (one way to infuse fluids, medicines, etc., into the body)

L

lateralis [L.]	(lăt´´ĕr-ā´lĭs)	a term denoting a structure situated farther from the midplane of the body
LDH		lactic dehydrogenase (a lab test done on blood)
Lowman turkey-claw clamp	(lō´măn)	orthopedic equipment used in surgery

M

MI		myocardial infarction
Micronase®	(mī´krō-nās)	trade name for glyburide; used in the management of non–insulin-dependent diabetes mellitus
myocardial	(mī´´ō-kăr´dē-ăl)	pertaining to the muscular tissue of the heart

N

Nitro-Dur®	(nī´tră dŭr)	trade name for nitroglycerin; used in treating angina pectoris and other cardiac problems
nondiaphoretic	(nŏn-dī´´ah-fō-rĕt´ĭk)	no profuse perspiration
normocephalic	(nōr´´mō-sĕ-făl´ĭk)	pertaining to a normal-sized head

O

OR		operating room
organomegaly	(ŏr´´gah-nō-mĕg´ă-lē)	enlargement of the viscera (internal organs)
ORIF		open reduction, internal fixation (of a fracture)

P

palpable	(păl´pah-b'l)	perceptible by touch
PERRLA		pupils equal, round, and reactive to light and accommodation
plane		a flat surface determined by the position of three points in space
PMI		point of maximal impulse (cardiac term)
prominence	(prŏm´ĭ-nĕns)	a protrusion or projection
prosthesis	(prŏs-thē´sĭs)	an artificial substitute for a missing body part, such as an eye, arm, or leg, used for either functional or cosmetic reasons
proximal		nearest; closer to any point of reference

R

reamer	(rē´mĕr)	an instrument used in orthopedic surgery to create a hollow area in bone
renal insufficiency		a state of disordered function of the kidneys verifiable by quantitative tests
rhonchus	(rŏng´kŭs)	a rattling in the throat; also a dry, coarse rale in the bronchial tubes, due to a partial obstruction (pl. rhonchi)
rub (pericardial rub)	(pĕr´´ĭ-kăr´dē-ăl rŭb)	a scraping or grating noise heard with the heartbeat

S

sclera	(sklē´rah)	the rough white outer coat of the eyeball (pl. sclerae)
SGOT		serum glutamic oxaloacetic transaminase (a lab test done on blood)
ST-T waves		how heart function is described on an electrocardiogram; there are P, Q, R, S, T, and U waves

T

TM		tympanic membrane (in the ear)
type and cross x 2		medical jargon referring to the fact that the patient's blood type needs to be determined by laboratory personnel, then crossmatched against 2 units of blood. This blood will be held for the patient if the patient needs it during surgery. If not, it will be released for crossmatch against another patient's blood.

U

UA		urinalysis (or urine analysis)

V

vastus [L.]	(văs´tŭs)	great or vast
Vicryl®	(vī´krĭl)	trade name for an absorbable suture

W

Wygesic®	(wī-jē´zĭk)	trade name for a pain medication

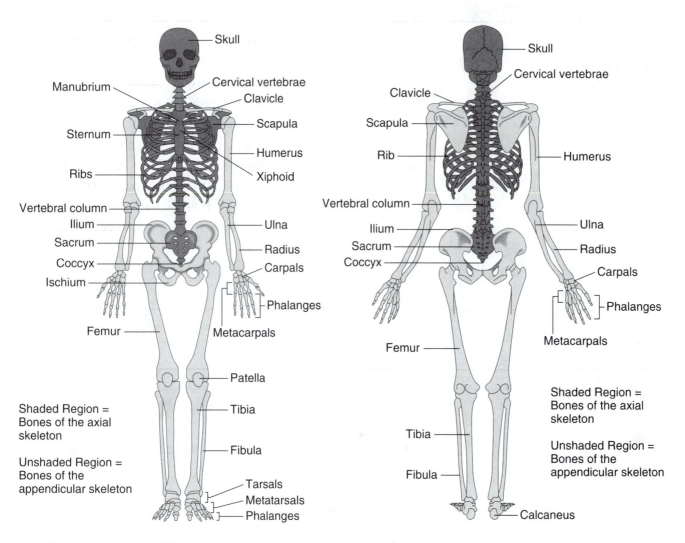

2.1 (A) Anterior view of the adult human skeleton.   (B) Posterior view of the adult human skeleton.

Case 3: The Cardiovascular System

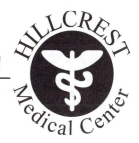

Patient Name

Steve Vaccaro

Address

3506 N.W. 56th Court
North Miami Beach, FL 33160-5938

Situation

Steve Vaccaro is an older man with a history of having fainted. He was brought in to the hospital emergency room to be evaluated. The patient was admitted to the intensive care unit by the emergency room physician. It was decided that a cardiologist was needed to perform an operative procedure on the patient, the implantation of a pacemaker. Mr. Vaccaro was kept in ICU until he stabilized and then was transferred to the floor of the hospital where cardiac patients are sent after surgery. After determining that the patient was suitably improved for discharge, the admitting physician discharged him to be followed in the office of the cardiologist.

Review Illustration 3-1, Structures of the Heart, and Illustration 3-2, AICDs, on page 93.

Student Name _____

Patient: Steve Vaccaro

Sequence of Reports	Date Completed	Grade
History and Physical Examination	_____	_____
Operative Report	_____	_____
Discharge Summary	_____	_____

Enter the date of completion for each report. When you have finished all reports, tear this sheet out, staple it to the front of the reports (in the order listed above), and give the completed reports to your instructor.

Glossary for Case 3
WORDS & PHONETIC PRONUNCIATIONS   DEFINITIONS

A

afebrile	(ā-fĕb´rĭl)	without fever
angina	(ăn-jī´nah) (ăn´jĕ-nah)	spasmodic, choking, or suffocating pain
atrial	(ā´trē-ăl)	pertaining to an atrium (chamber) of the heart

B

bilateral	(bī-lăt´ĕr-ăl)	pertaining to both sides

C

C&S		culture and sensitivity (done in the lab)
cardiomegaly	(kăr´´dē-ō-mĕg´ah-lē)	enlargement of the heart
Chem-20		chemical profile resulting in 20 different values (done on either blood or serum)
clubbing		a growing change (broadening) of the soft tissues around the ends of the fingers or toes; the nails are abnormally curved and shiny
cyanosis	(sī´´ah-nō´sĭs)	a bluish discoloration

D

Darvocet-N®	(dăr´vō-sĕt ĕn)	narcotic analgesic drug (trade name)
deviated septum		usually relating to a nose with the dividing wall (septum) in the wrong place by either congenital anomaly or trauma; surgical correction is necessary
diaphoresis	(dī´´ah-fō-rē´sĭs)	profuse perspiration

| digoxin | (dī-jŏks´ĭn) | digitalis-type drug for congestive heart failure |

E

| ectopy | (ĕk´tō-pē) | displacement or malposition, especially if congenital |

F

| fibrillation | (fī´´brĭ-lă´shŭn) | a small, local, involuntary contraction of muscle, invisible under the skin, resulting from spontaneous activation of single muscle cells or muscle fibers |

H

hematocrit (Hct)	(hē-măt´ō-krĭt)	the volume percentage of erythrocytes in whole blood
hematoma	(hēm´´ah-tō´mah)	a localized collection of blood, usually clotted, in an organ, space, or tissue, due to a break in the wall of a blood vessel
hemoglobin (Hgb)	(hē´´mō-glō´bĭn)	the oxygen-carrying pigment of the erythrocytes, formed by the developing erythrocyte in bone marrow
hepatitis	(hĕp´´ah-tī´tĭs)	inflammation of the liver
histoplasmosis	(hĭs´´tō-plăz-mō´sĭs)	infection resulting from inhalation or, infrequently, the ingestion of spores of *Histoplasma capsulatum*
hypercholesterolemia	(hī´´pĕr-kō-lĕs´´tĕr-ŏl-ē´mē-ah)	excess cholesterol in the blood
hyperlipidemia	(hī´´pĕr-lĭp´´ĭ-dē´mē-ah)	a general term for elevated concentrations of any or all of the lipids (fats) in the plasma
hypertension	(hī´´pĕr-tĕn´shŭn)	persistently high arterial blood pressure
hypertrophy	(hī-pĕr´trō-fē)	the enlargement or overgrowth of an organ

hypomagnesemia	(hī´´pō-măg´´nē-sē´mē-ah)	an abnormally low magnesium content of the blood plasma

I

ICU		intensive care unit
I&O		intake and output (sometimes dictated as "ins and outs")
isoenzyme	(ī´´sō-ĕn´zīm)	a tumor-associated antigen

J

JVD		jugular venous distention (in the neck)

L

Lanoxin®	(lah-nŏk´sĭn)	digitalis-type drug for congestive heart failure (trade name)
lateral	(lăt´ĕr-ăl)	pertaining to a side
lidocaine	(lī´dō-kān)	used as a topical anesthetic or as a spinal anesthetic; can also be used as an antiarrhythmic drug
Lopressor®	(lō-prĕs´ŏr)	drug used for hypertension and angina (trade name)
lorazepam	(lŏr-ah´zĕ-păm)	antianxiety drug
lymphadenopathy	(lĭm-făd´´ĕ-nŏp´ah-thē)	any disease process affecting the lymph node(s)

M

myocardial infarction (MI)	(mī´´ō-kăr´dē-ăl ĭn-fărk´shŭn)	gross necrosis of the myocardium as a result of interruption of the blood supply to the area

N

nephrolithiasis	(nĕf´´rō-lĭ-thī´ah-sĭs)	a condition marked by the presence of renal calculi

niacin		nonprescription dietary supplement used to treat hypercholesterolemia (nicotinic acid)
nitroglycerin	(nī-trō-glĭs´ĕr-ĭn)	antianginal drug (generic)
Nitrostat®	(nī´trō-stăt)	antianginal drug, usually taken sublingually (trade name)

O

orthopnea	(ŏr˝thŏp-nē´ah)	difficult breathing except in an upright position or while using several pillows, e.g., 3-pillow orthopnea

P

PAC		premature atrial contraction (a cardiac term)
paresthesia	(păr˝ĕs-thē´zē-ah)	an abnormal sensation, as burning or prickling
paroxysm	(păr´ŏk-sĭzm)	a sudden recurrence or intensification of symptoms
periarteritis nodosa	(pĕr˝ē-ăr˝tĕ-rī´tĭs nō-dō´sah)	an inflammatory disease of the coats of the small and medium-sized arteries of the body, associated with a variety of systemic symptoms
periorbital	(pĕr˝ē-ŏr´bĭ-tăl)	situated around the orbit or eye socket
polypectomy	(pŏl˝ĭ-pĕk´tō-mē)	surgical removal of a polyp
posteroanterior (PA)	(pŏs˝tĕr-ō-ăn-tēr´ē-ŏr)	pertaining to the direction from back to front
PVC		premature ventricular contraction (a cardiac term)

Q

Quinaglute®	(kwĭn´ah-glūte)	antiarrhythmic drug (trade name)
quinidine	(kwĭn´ĭ-dĭn)	antiarrhythmic drug (generic)

S

subclavian	(sŭb-klā′vē-ăn)	situated under the clavicle
sublingual	(sŭb-lĭng′gwăl)	located beneath the tongue
superior vena cava	(ve′nah kā′vah)	the venous trunk draining blood from the head, neck, upper extremities, and chest
syncope	(sĭn′kō-pē)	a brief loss of consciousness; fainting
synovectomy	(sĭn″ō-vĕk′tō-mē)	removal of a synovial membrane

T

tachybradycardia	(tăk″ē-brăd″ē-kar′dē-ah)	fast and slow heartbeat
thrombosis	(thrŏm-bō′sĭs)	formation or presence of a thrombus or blood clot
thyromegaly	(thī″rō-mĕg′ah-lē)	enlargement of the thyroid gland
transvenous	(trăns-vē′nŭs)	performed through a vein
TSH		thyroid-stimulating hormone (a lab test)
turgor	(tŭr′gŏr)	swollen and congested

U

urinalysis (UA)	(ū″rĭ-năl′ĭ-sĭs)	physical, chemical, or microscopic analysis or examination of urine

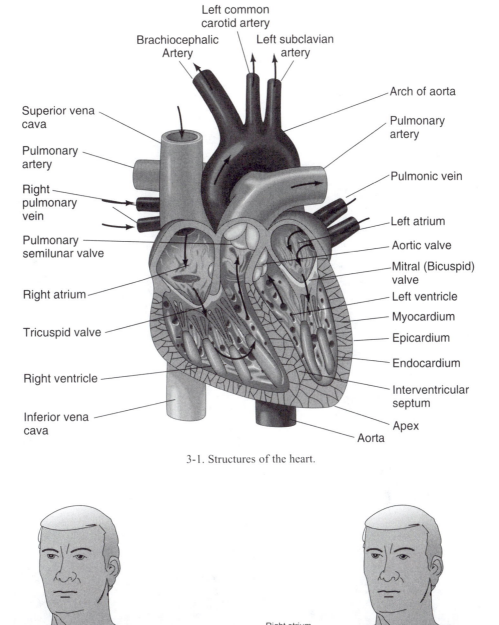

3-1. Structures of the heart.

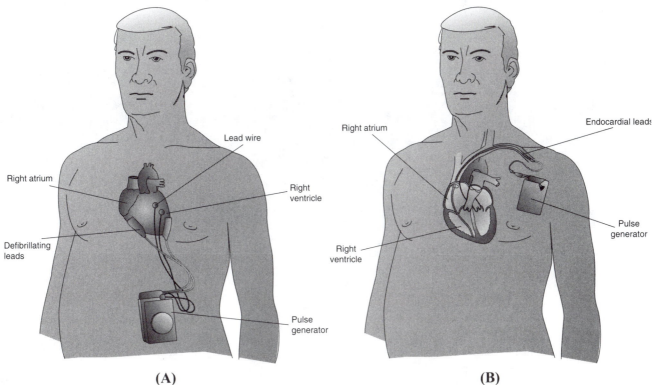

(A)   **(B)**

3-2. Two different types of automatic implantable cardioverter-defibrillators (AICD). (A) AICD has pulse generator implanted in the sub-cutaneous tissue of the abdomen with lead wires and a defibrillating lead going to the heart. (B) AICD with pulse generator implanted below the collarbone with endocardial leads positioned in the heart through a vein.

Case 4: The Integumentary System

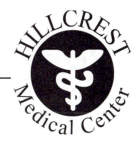

Patient Name

Gloria Ramos

Address

5900 S.E. 22nd Avenue
Miami Beach, FL 33156-5937

Situation

Gloria Ramos is a middle-aged woman with multiple medical problems who developed painful ulcerations of her mouth and lips, making eating and drinking difficult. She sought medical treatment at her internist's office for her problem, and he admitted her to Hillcrest Medical Center. Ms. Ramos had a routine chest x-ray on admission, and she was referred to dermatology services in consultation. The dermatologist and internist agreed on a treatment plan for the patient, and after a few days marked improvement was noted in her condition. She was discharged in improved condition to be followed by the internist and the dermatologist as needed.

Review Illustration 4-1, Anatomy of the Skin, on page 101.

Student Name _____

Patient: Gloria Ramos

Sequence of Reports	Date Completed	Grade
History and Physical Examination	_____	_____
Radiology Report	_____	_____
Request for Consultation	_____	_____
Discharge Summary	_____	_____

Enter the date of completion for each report. When you have finished all reports, tear this sheet out, staple it to the front of the reports (in the order listed above), and give the completed reports to your instructor.

Glossary for Case 4

WORDS & PHONETIC PRONUNCIATIONS   DEFINITIONS

A

albeit	(ăl-bē´ĭt)	even though
albumin	(ăl-bū´mĭn)	a necessary protein substance produced in the liver; levels are reduced in malnutrition and in hepatic and renal diseases
arthritis	(ăr-thrī´tĭs)	inflammation of the joints
azathioprine	(ā´zah-thī´ō-prēn)	generic drug used in treating rheumatoid arthritis and other autoimmune diseases
Azulfidine®	(ā-zŭl´fĭ-dēn)	trade name for sulfasalazine, an antibacterial agent

C

chlorambucil	(klō-răm´bū-sĭl)	generic drug, an antineoplastic agent
compression fracture	(kŏr´´tĭ-kō-stē´roids)	any break or rupture of bone due to compression, for example, the bones in the spinal cord
corticosteroids		a group of steroids (or lipids) used clinically to suppress the immune response and in hormonal replacement, etc.
cyclophosphamide	(sī´´klō-fŏs´fah-mīd)	generic drug, an antineoplastic agent

D

debilitating		causing a loss or lack of strength
dehydration	(dē´´hī-drā´shŭn)	condition resulting from excess loss of body water
dermatology	(dĕr´´mah-tŏl´ō-jē)	the study of the skin

diffuse	(dĭ-fūs´)	widely distributed; to pass through or spread widely through a tissue or structure
Disalcid®	(dī-săl´sĭd)	a nonsteroidal anti-inflammatory drug used to treat minor pain, fever, and arthritis (trade name)
distally	(dĭs´tăl-lē)	in a distal or remote direction; opposite of proximal or near
Dolobid®	(dō´lō-bĭd)	trade name for diflunisal; used to treat mild to moderate pain
dysphagia	(dĭs-fā´jē-ah)	difficulty in swallowing

E

ecchymosis	(ĕk´´ĭ-mō´sĭs)	a small spot on the skin or mucous membrane forming a nonelevated, rounded or irregular, blue or purplish patch (pl. ecchymoses)
enteritis	(ĕn´´tĕr-ī´tĭs)	inflammation of the intestine, particularly the small intestine
erosion	(ē-rō´zhŭn)	a gradual breakdown or very shallow ulceration of the skin; destruction of the surface of a tissue
erythema	(ĕr´´ĭ-thē´mah)	redness of the skin produced by congestion of the capillaries
erythema multiforme	(mŭl´tĭ-fŏrm´´āy)	a symptom complex including multiple skin lesions of a varying degree of severity
etiology	(ē´´tē-ŏl´ō´jē)	cause or origin of a disease or disorder
exophthalmos	(ĕk´´sŏf-thăl´mōs)	abnormal protrusion of the eyeball
exudate	(ĕks´ū-dāt)	material such as fluid, cells, or cellular debris that has escaped from blood vessels and been deposited in tissues, usually as a result of inflammation

F

fissuring	(fĭsh´ūr-ĭng)	splitting, normal or otherwise; can include painful ulcerations
folic acid	(fō´lĭk ăs´ĭd)	a B complex vitamin, the lack of which can result in severe anemia

G

gingiva	(jĭn´jĭ-vah)	the pale pink tissues of the oral mucosa, otherwise known as the gums

H

HCTZ		abbreviation for hydrochlorothiazide, a generic drug; a diuretic used to treat edema and hypertension
hydroxychloroquine	(hī-drŏk´´sē-klō´rō-kwĭn)	generic drug used to treat rheumatoid arthritis
hyperpigmentation	(hī´´pĕr-pĭg´´mĕn-tā´shŭn)	abnormally increased coloration
hyporeflexia	(hī´pō-rē-flĕk´sē-ah)	weakness of the reflexes

I

IV hydration		receiving fluids intravenously
injection (noun)		the condition of being injected or congested or overloaded with blood
intravenous	(ĭn´´trah-vē´nŭs)	within a vein

K

kyphosis	(kī-fō´sĭs)	abnormally increased curvature of thoracic spine; humpback

L

leucovorin	(loo´´kō-vō´rĭn)	generic drug used to treat both anemia and malignancies

Lidex® gel	(lī′dĕks jĕl)	trade name for a topically applied gel; an anti-inflammatory agent
liver enzymes	(lĭv′ĕr ĕn′zīms)	those protein molecules that induce necessary chemical reactions in the liver; the group of laboratory tests on blood or serum that give the values of these proteins

M

macular	(măk′ū-lăr)	pertaining to the presence of a macule, a discolored spot on the skin not elevated above the surface
malaise	(măl-āz′)	a vague feeling of bodily discomfort
methotrexate		generic drug, an antineoplastic agent; also used in immunosuppressive disorders

N

nephrocalcinosis	(nĕf′′rō-kăl′′sĭ-nō′sĭs)	diffusely scattered calcifications in the kidneys leading to renal insufficiency
NSAID		abbreviation for nonsteroidal anti-inflammatory drug

O

osteoporosis	(ŏs′′tē-ō-pō-rō′sĭs)	reduction in the amount of bone mass leading to fractures after minimal trauma

P

penicillamine	(pĕn′′ĭ-sĭl′ah-mēn)	generic drug, a product of penicillin; used to treat rheumatoid arthritis
perimalleolar	(pĕr′′ĭ-măl-ē′ō-lăr)	around the bony protuberances on either side of the ankle

pitting edema		when too much fluid is in the tissues (edema) and the finger pressing on the skin leaves pitting indentations in the skin
p.o. [L.]	(pĕr ŏs)	by mouth (per os)
posterior pharynx	(făr´ĭnks)	the back of the throat
prednisone	(prĕd´nĭ-sōn)	generic drug, an anti-inflammatory agent
Premarin®	(prēm´ah-rĭn)	trade name for preparations of estrogen, the female hormone

Q

q.o.d.		every other day (not Latin, but more jargon)
quiescent		at rest; inactive

R

regimen	(rĕj´ĭ-mĕn)	a strictly regulated scheme of therapy, diet, exercise, or other activity designed to achieve a certain goal
rheumatoid arthritis	(roo´mah-toid ăr-thrī´tĭs)	chronic systemic, painful joint disease that can result in deformities; cause unknown

S

serum cholesterol	(sē´rŭm kō-lĕs´tĕr-ŏl)	the level of cholesterol (a complex organic compound synthesized in the liver and other tissues) found in the serum; high levels of cholesterol can both clog arteries and form gallstones
stasis edema	(stā´sĭs ĕ-dē´mah)	stagnation of the flow of blood or fluids
Stevens-Johnson syndrome		a severe, sometimes fatal multisystemic form of erythema multiforme

stomatitis	(stō-mah-tī´tĭs)	inflammation of the oral mucosa

T

t.i.d. [L.]		(ter in die) three times a day
topically		referring to a surface area; applying a substance to a certain surface area of the skin
total protein		a laboratory test to determine the level of all proteins in the serum

V

vertebral bodies	(vĕr´tĕ-brăl) (vĕr-tē´brăl)	any of the 33 bones of the spinal canal
volume depletion		dehydrated state

W

Westergren sedimentation rate		standard laboratory test to determine the erythrocyte sedimentation rate (ESR) using a tube and a method designed by Dr. Westergren

4-1. Anatomy of the skin.

Case 5: The Urinary System

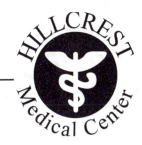

Patient Name

Carlos Lopez

Address

509 Red Road
Miami, FL 33114-0229

Situation

Carlos Lopez is an elderly patient who has suffered with difficulty emptying his urinary bladder. He went to his family physician, who referred him to a urologist, a surgeon specializing in the treatment of the urinary tract and the male genitalia. The patient was taken to surgery to solve his problem, and the tissues removed were sent to a pathologist for both macroscopic and microscopic examination and diagnosis. The patient was subsequently discharged from the hospital by his family physician, to be followed as an outpatient by both the family physician and the urologist.

Review Illustration 5-1 A and B, The Urinary System, and Cross-section of the Kidney, on page 109.

Student Name _____

Patient: Carlos Lopez

Sequence of Reports	Date Completed	Grade
History and Physical Examination	_____	_____
Operative Report	_____	_____
Pathology Report	_____	_____
Discharge Summary	_____	_____

Enter the date of completion for each report. When you have finished all reports, tear this sheet out, staple it to the front of the reports (in the order listed above), and give the completed reports to your instructor.

Glossary for Case 5

WORDS & PHONETIC PRONUNCIATIONS   DEFINITIONS

A

atrophy	(ăt´rō-fē)	a wasting away; a diminution in the size of a cell, tissue, organ, or part
autonomic	(aw´´tō-nŏm´ĭk)	self-controlling; functionally independent

B

Bactrim DS®	(băk´trĭm)	combination antibiotic and sulfonamide anti-infective; this drug is used for urinary tract, respiratory tract, and ear infections (trade name)
bruit [Fr.]	(brwē) (bro͞ot)	a sound or murmur heard on auscultation, especially an abnormal one; usually used in the plural, bruits
BUN		blood urea nitrogen (a lab test done on blood)

C

carotid	(kah-rŏt´ĭd)	relating to the principal artery of the neck
CBC		complete blood count
cholecystectomy	(kō´´lē-sĭs-tĕk´tō-mē)	surgical removal of the gallbladder
corpora amylacea [L.]	(kŏr´pō-rah ăm´´ĭ-lā´sē-ah)	small hyaline masses of degenerate cells found in the prostate (sing. corpus amylaceum)
creatinine	(krē-ăt´ĭ-nĭn)	the end product of creatine metabolism, found in muscle and blood and excreted in the urine
CT		computed tomography (a radiology procedure)

cystourethroscope	(sĭs´´tō-ū-rē´thrō-skōp)	an instrument for examining the bladder and posterior urethra
cystourethroscopy	(sĭs´´tō-ū´´rē-thrŏs´ko̅-pē)	process of visually examining the bladder and posterior urethra

D
_____

diverticulum	(dī´´vĕr-tĭk´ū-lŭm)	a circumscribed pouch or sac of variable size occurring normally or created by herniation of the lining mucous membrane through a defect in the muscular coat of a tubular organ, like the colon (pl. diverticula)
dysuria	(dĭs-ū´rē-ah)	painful or difficult urination

E
_____

efflux	(ĕf´lŭks)	a flowing out or emanating
electrocardiogram (EKG)	(ē-lĕk´´trō-kăr´dē-ō-grăm´´)	a graphic tracing of the variations in electrical potential caused by the excitation of the heart muscle and detected at the body surface (sometimes abbreviated ECG)

F
_____

Foley catheter	(fō´lē kăth´ĕ-tĕr)	an indwelling catheter retained in the bladder by a balloon, which may be inflated with air or liquid
French scale		a scale used for denoting the size of catheters, sounds, and other tubular instruments, each unit being roughly equivalent to 0.33 mm in diameter

G
_____

gastrointestinal (GI)	(găs´´trō-ĭn-tĕs´tĭ-năl)	pertaining to the stomach and intestine
granuloma	(grăn´´ū-lō´mah)	a tumor-like mass or nodule of granulation tissue

granulomatous	(grăn″ū-lŏm′ah-tŭs)	composed of granulomas

H

HEENT		head, eyes, ears, nose, throat
hematuria	(hēm″ah-tū′rē-ah)	blood in the urine
hyperplasia	(hī″pĕr-plā′zē-ah)	an abnormal increase in the number of normal cells in normal arrangement in a tissue
hypotension	(hī″pō-tĕn′shŭn)	abnormally low blood pressure
Hytrin®	(hī′trĭn)	antihypertensive drug (trade name)

I

induration	(ĭn′dū-rā′shŭn)	The quality of being hard; the process of hardening
indwell		to dwell in; reside within

L

lithiasis	(lĭ-thī′ah-sĭs)	the formation of calculi or mineral concretions within the body
lithotomy	(lĭ-thŏt′ō-mē)	incision of a duct or organ, especially of the urinary bladder, for removal of stone(s)

O

optic fundi	(ŏp′tĭk fŭn′dī)	pertaining to the base of the eyes
orifice	(ŏr′ĭ-fĭs)	the entrance or outlet of any cavity in the body
orthostatic	(ŏr″thō-stăt′ĭk)	pertaining to or caused by standing erect

P

prostate	(prŏs´tāt)	a gland in the male that surrounds the neck of the urinary bladder and the urethra
prothrombin	(prō-thrŏm´bĭn)	a factor in the blood plasma that combines with calcium to form thrombin during blood clotting
PTT		partial thromboplastin time; one test to determine how fast the blood clots

R

rale [Fr.]	(rahl)	an abnormal respiratory sound heard on auscultation, indicating some pathologic condition
renal	(rē´năl)	pertaining to the kidney
resect	(rē-sĕkt´)	to remove part of an organ or tissue
resectoscope	(rē-sĕk´tō-skōp)	an instrument with a wide-angle telescope and an electrically activated wire loop for transurethral removal or biopsy of lesions of the bladder, prostate, or urethra

S

sphincter	(sfĭngk´tĕr)	a ringlike band of muscle fibers that either constricts a passage or closes a natural orifice
splenomegaly	(splē´´nō-mĕg´ah-lē)	enlargement of the spleen
stroma	(strō´mah)	the supporting tissue of an organ, as distinguished from its functional element

T

trabeculate	(trah-bĕk´ū-lāt)	marked with cross bars
trabeculation	(trah-bĕk´´ū-lā´shŭn)	the formation of trabeculae in a part

trachea	(trā´kē-ah)	the cartilaginous and membranous tube descending from the larynx and branching into the right and left main bronchi
transurethral resection (TUR)	(trăns´´ū-rē´thrăl rē-sĕk´shŭn)	a surgical procedure to relieve urinary obstruction by reaming out the enlarged part of the gland that is encroaching on the urethra and blocking outflow of urine

V

void		to cast out as waste matter

W

wheeze		an abnormal whistling sound made in breathing

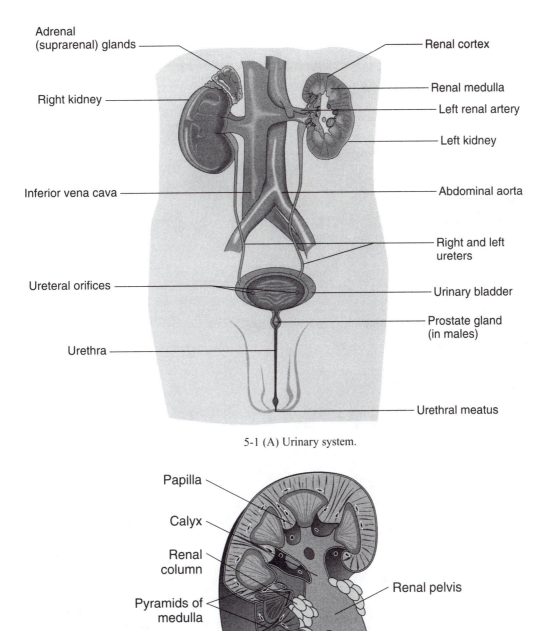

5-1 (A) Urinary system.

5-1 (B) Cross-section of the kidney.

Case 6: The Nervous System

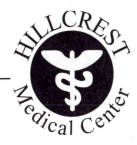

Patient Name

Lydia Cruz

Address

7334 Kendall Avenue
Miami, FL 33156-5948

Situation

After suffering with long-term pain in both her low back and right leg and receiving no benefit from chiropractic manipulation, Mrs. Cruz sought advice and treatment from a neurosurgeon. She was admitted to Hillcrest for radiology testing, which revealed her to have a herniated disc. She was taken to surgery where the herniated disc was removed and the tissue sent to pathology for examination and diagnosis. After an uneventful, afebrile hospital course, the patient was discharged in improved condition, with her pain resolved.

Review Illustration 6-1, Spinal Column, and Illustration 6-2, Intervertebral/herniated discs, on page 117.

Student Name _____

Patient: Lydia Cruz

Sequence of Reports	Date Completed	Grade
History and Physical Examination	_____	_____
Radiology Report x 2	_____	_____
Operative Report	_____	_____
Pathology Report	_____	_____
Discharge Summary	_____	_____

Enter the date of completion for each report. When you have finished all reports, tear this sheet out, staple it to the front of the reports (in the order listed above), and give the completed reports to your instructor.

Glossary for Case 6
WORDS & PHONETIC PRONUNCIATIONS   DEFINITIONS

Word & Pronunciation	Definition
2 + knee and ankle jerks	this phrase refers to the sudden reflex or involuntary movements made when the doctor is examining the knees and ankles; part of the neurologic exam; in this case they are graded as 2 +, which means average

A

Word & Pronunciation	Definition
aggregating	crowding or clustering together
ambulating (ăm´´bū-lā´tīng)	walking
arthropathy (ăr-thrŏp´ah-thē)	any joint disease

B

Word & Pronunciation	Definition
blunted	to make less sharp or defined; dull

C

Word & Pronunciation	Definition
cesarean (sē-sār´ē-ăn)	referring to cesarean section, an incision through the abdominal and uterine walls for delivery of a fetus
chiropractor (kī´´rō-prăk´tŏr)	a practitioner of chiropractic, a conservative science of applied neurophysiology; e.g., chiropractors believe irritation of the nervous system is the cause of disease
Cloward saddle (klow´ĕrd)	surgical equipment in which a patient is placed for back fusion
contrast medium	a substance that is introduced into or around a structure and, because of the difference in absorption of x-rays by both the contrast medium and the surrounding tissues, allows radiographic

		visualization of the structure (pl. contrast media)
contused	(kŏn-tūzd´)	bruised
convex	(kŏn´vĕks)	having a rounded, somewhat elevated surface
curette	(kū-rĕt´)	spoon-shaped instrument for removing material from the wall of a cavity or other surface

D

Darvocet®	(dăr´vō-sĕt)	trade name for drug used to treat mild to moderate pain
denies x 3		this phrase, as used in the Social History, refers to the fact that the patient denies alcohol, tobacco, and illicit drug use
discectomy	(dĭs-kĕk´tō-mē)	excision of an intervertebral disc
discrete		made up of separated parts or characterized by lesions that do not become blended

E

epinephrine	(ĕp´´ĭ-nĕf´rĭn)	generic drug used as a vasoconstrictor, cardiac stimulant, and bronchodilator; also called adrenaline
exacerbate	(ĕg-zăs´ĕr-bāt´´)	to increase in severity

F

facet	(făs´ĕt)	a small plane surface on a hard body, as on a bone
Flexeril®	(flĕks´ĕr-ĭl)	trade name for drug used to treat muscle spasm
focal degeneration		main area or center of deterioration

formalin	(fŏr´mah-lĭn)	a powerful disinfectant gas, used in water as a fluid to preserve tissue removed at surgery for pathologic evaluation; same as formaldehyde

G

Gelfoam® sponge		trade name for absorbable gelatin sponge; sterile, they are used in surgery to stop the flow of blood
gutter		low area, trough, or groove

H

herniated	(hĕr´nē-āt´´ĕd)	protruding like a hernia; enclosed in a hernia

I

i.e. [L.]		(id est) that is
intermittent		occurring at separated intervals; having periods of cessation of activity
intervertebral	(ĭn´´tĕr-vĕr´tĕ-brăl) (ĭn´´tĕr-vĕrtē´brăl)	situated between two contiguous vertebrae

K

Kantrex®	(kăn´trĕks)	trade name for an antibiotic

L

L1-2		lumbar spine, between first and second vertebrae (the disc space)
L2-3		lumbar spine, between second and third vertebrae (the disc space)
L3-4		lumbar spine, between third and fourth vertebrae (the disc space)
L4-5		lumbar spine, between fourth and fifth vertebrae (the disc space)

L5/S1 or L5-S1		lumbar spine, fifth vertebra, and sacral spine, first vertebra (where the lumbar and sacral spines join)
lamina	(lăm´ĭ-nah)	a thin, flat plate or layer
laminectomy	(lăm´´ĭ-něk´tō-mē)	excision of the posterior arch of a vertebra
lateral recess syndrome		A small hollow or indentation on the side of the fourth ventricle; by way of this recess part of the fourth ventricle protrudes into the subarachnoid space
ligamentum flavum [L.]	(lĭg´´ah-měn´tŭm flāv´ŭm)	band of yellow elastic tissue that assists in maintaining or regaining the erect position
light touch		when the doctor lightly strokes a part of the body, such as the extremities, to determine the patient's ability to feel; used in evaluation of the central nervous system
lumbosacral	(lŭm´´bō-sā´krăl)	pertaining to the loins and sacrum

M

Marcaine®	(măr-kān´)	trade name for local, injectable anesthetic agent
MVA		motor vehicle accident
myelogram	(mī´ĕ-lō-grăm)	an x-ray of the spinal cord

N

Norflex®	(nŏr´flĕks)	trade name for a drug used to treat muscle spasms

P

PAR		postanesthesia recovery; where patients are sent immediately after surgery

pinprick		when the doctor actually pricks a patient's skin with a sharp point to determine the level of feeling; part of the evaluation of the central nervous system
pleura	(ploor´ah)	a serous membrane lining the thoracic cavity, also known as the pleural cavity
prone	(prōn)	lying face downward

R

radicular	(rah-dĭk´ū-lăr)	of or pertaining to a radical, i.e., directed to the cause or root of a morbid process, such as radical surgery
retraction		the act of drawing back; the condition of being drawn back
rongeur [Fr.]	(raw-zhŭr´)	an instrument for cutting tough tissue, particularly bone

S

S1 root		sacral spine, first vertebra, at the lowest part
sacroiliac	(sā´´krō-ĭl´ē-ăk)	the sacral and iliac spines; where they join and their associated ligaments
scaphoid	(skăf´oid)	shaped like a boat; the scaphoid bone
scoliosis	(skō´´lē-ō´sĭs)	a sideways deviation in the normally straight vertical line of the spine (S-shaped spine)
spurring		projecting bodies, as from a bone
straight-leg raising		the doctor observes the patient's ability to raise the legs; part of the evaluation of the central nervous system
subarachnoid space	(sŭb´´ah-răk´noid spās)	space under the arachnoid membrane, between it and the pia mater

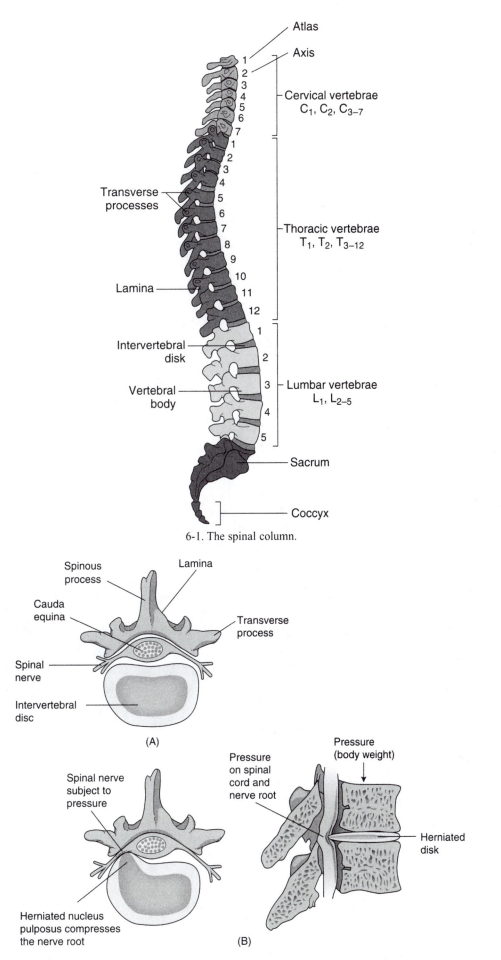

6-1. The spinal column.

(A)

(B)

6-2. (A)Normal intervertebral disc. (B) Two views of a herniated disc.

Case 7: The Digestive System

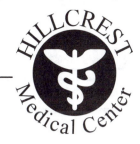

Patient Name

Janice McClure

Address

10620 S.W. 72nd Court
Miami, FL 33156-5902

Situation

This elderly female had been suffering from acute abdominal pain for a few weeks before she finally presented to the Hillcrest emergency room for treatment. The emergency room physician examined her, ordered x-ray studies, admitted her, and referred her to a surgeon for evaluation. The consulting surgeon reviewed the x-ray findings, examined the patient, and discussed the patient's options with her and her family. They agreed on surgery as soon as possible, which was carried out that day. An x-ray was done during the surgical procedure, and the tissues removed at surgery were submitted to pathology for gross and microscopic description and diagnosis. After an uneventful postoperative course, the patient was discharged to follow-up with the surgeon in 2 days.

Review Illustration 7-1, The Digestive System, on page 127.

Student Name _____

Patient: Janice McClure

Sequence of Reports	Date Completed	Grade
History and Physical Examination	_____	_____
Request for Consultation	_____	_____
Operative Report	_____	_____
Radiology Report	_____	_____
Pathology Report	_____	_____
Discharge Summary	_____	_____

Enter the date of completion for each report. When you have finished all reports, tear this sheet out, staple it to the front of the reports (in the order listed above), and give the completed reports to your instructor.

Glossary for Case 7

WORDS & PHONETIC PRONUNCIATIONS		DEFINITIONS

A

adenopathy	(ăd´´ĕ-nŏp´ah-thē)	enlargement of the glands, especially the lymphatic glands
amoxicillin	(ah-mŏks´´ĭ-sĭl´ĭn)	generic antibiotic used against a wide variety of bacteria
ampulla	(ăm-pŭl´lah)	a pouched dilatation or enlargement of a canal or duct
atypia	(ā-tĭp´ē-ah)	the condition of being irregular, not conforming to type

B

bilirubin	(bĭl´´ĭ-roo´bĭn)	a bile pigment circulating in plasma

C

calcification	(kăl´´sĭ-fĭ-kā´shŭn)	the process by which organic tissue becomes hardened by a deposit of calcium salts
cholecystitis	(kō´´lē-sĭs-tī´tĭs)	inflammation of the gallbladder
choledocholithiasis	(kō-lĕd´´ō-kō-lĭ-thī´ah-sĭs)	the occurrence of calculi (stones) in the common bile duct
choledocholithotomy	(kō-lĕd´´ō-kō-lĭ-thŏt´ō-mē)	incision of the common bile duct for the removal of stone(s)
choledochoscopy	(kō-lĕd´´ō-kŏs´kō-pē)	examination of the interior of the common bile duct (by instrument)
cholelithiasis	(kō´´lē-lĭ-thī´ah-sĭs)	the presence or formation of gallstones
clips		surgical equipment; metallic devices for holding closed the edges of a wound

common bile duct		one of the ducts conveying bile in and from the liver to the small intestine
cranial nerves II through XII		referred to by Roman numerals, the twelve pairs of nerves connected with the brain; cranial nerve I (olfactory) is traditionally not included in the routine physical examination
cystic artery	(sĭs´tĭk ăr´tĕr-ē)	the artery that originates in the right branch of the hepatic (liver) artery and goes to the gallbladder

D

dentition	(dĕn-tĭsh´ŭn)	the natural teeth in the dental arch
dilatation	(dĭl-ah-tā´shŭn)	the condition of being stretched beyond normal dimensions; the act of stretching
diplopia	(dĭplō´pē-ah)	the perception of two images of a single object (seeing double)
duodenum	(dū´´ō-dē´nŭm) (dū-ŏd´ĕ-nŭm)	the first portion of the small intestine

E

emesis	(ĕm´ĕ-sĭs)	vomiting or the product derived from vomiting
eosinophils	(ē´´ō-sĭn´ō-fĭls)	cells readily stained by eosin (a red dye); part of what is reported on the differential cell count (often dictated as "eos")
ERCP		endoscopic retrograde cholangiopancreatography (an internal examination done in radiology)
expulsion		the act of expelling, driving, or forcing out
exquisite		extremely intense, sharp, as in exquisite pain or tenderness

F

fibrous tissue		tissue composed of or containing fibers, which are elongated, threadlike structures
filling defect		any localized defect in the contour of the stomach, duodenum, or intestine as seen on the x-ray after a barium enema; this filling defect would be due to either a lesion or an object in the contour
flatus	(flā′tŭs)	the gas or air normally in the gastrointestinal tract
follicular	(fō-lĭk′ū-lăr)	of or pertaining to a follicle or follicles (pouchlike depression or cavity)
frequency		the number of occurrences of a particular event, specifically urination at short intervals due to a reduced urinary bladder capacity

G

gallstones		concretions formed in the gallbladder or bile duct
GGT		gamma-glutamyl transpeptidase (lab test on blood)
GPT		glutamic-pyruvic transaminase (lab test on blood)
grossly		visible to the naked eye
guarding		a spasm of muscles to minimize motion or agitation of an injured or diseased site

H

hematemesis	(hĕm″ah-tĕm′ĕ-sĭs)	the vomiting of blood
hemoptysis	(hē-mŏp′tĭ-sĭs)	the expectoration of blood or blood-stained sputum

hepatosplenomegaly	(hĕp´´ah-tō-splē´nō-mĕg´ah-lē)	enlargement of the liver and spleen
hernia	(hĕr´nē-ah)	the protrusion of a loop or knuckle of an organ or tissue through an abnormal opening (pl. herniae or hernias)
hesitancy		an involuntary delay (or inability) in starting the urinary stream
HIV protocol		an explicit, detailed plan regarding protection of both health care workers and patients from the human immunodeficiency virus in the workplace

I

indices		plural of index; a guide, standard, or symbol
interrupted 1-O Novafil	(nō´vah-fĭl)	suture material used in the fashion whereby each stitch is made with a separate piece of material; the "one-O" indicates the thickness of the thread
intraoperative cholangiogram	(ĭn´´trah-ŏp´ĕr-ah´´tĭv kō-lăn´jē-ō-grăm´´)	an x-ray of the gallbladder and bile ducts done while the patient is actually undergoing surgery

J

Jackson-Pratt drain		a specific tool used in surgery to draw off fluid from a cavity as it forms (sometimes dictated as J-P drain)

K

Kocher clamp	(kō´kĕr)	a heavy, straight surgical instrument with interlocking teeth on the tip

L

laparoscopic cholecystectomy	(lăp´´ah-rō-skŏp´ĭk kō´´lē-sĭs-tĕk´tō-mē)	surgical removal of the gallbladder using an instrument (laparoscope) that, when inserted, allows examination, inspection, or removal; no incision is required ("lap chole" may be dictated)
lymphs	(lĭmfs)	acceptable medical jargon; shortened version of lymphocytes, which are white blood cells found in blood or lymph; a part of the differential white blood cell count

M

mammogram	(măm´ō-grăm)	an x-ray of the breast(s)
melena	(mĕl´ĕ-nă)	the passage of dark, blood-stained stool; black vomit
microbiology		the science that deals with the study of algae, bacteria, fungi, protozoa, and viruses
migraine	(mī´grān)	severe vascular headache
monos		acceptable medical jargon; shortened version of monocytes, which are white blood cells; a part of the differential white blood cell count
multiparous	(mŭl-tĭp´ah-rŭs)	having had two or more pregnancies that resulted in birth, live or not

N

n.p.o [L.]		nothing by mouth (per os)
needle-stick protocol		an explicit, detailed plan regarding the prevention of contaminated needle sticks to health care workers in the workplace
normocytic	(nŏr´´mō-sĭt´ĭk)	relating to or having the characteristics of a red blood cell that is normal in size, shape, and color

O

| open cholecystectomy | (ko´´lē-sĭs-tĕk´tō-mē) | a standard surgical procedure, including an incision, for the removal of the gallbladder; it refers to surgically opening the abdomen rather than using the laparoscopic procedure |

P

palpitations	(păl´´pĭ-tā´shŭnz)	sensation of unduly rapid or irregular heartbeat (should be used in the plural, even if dictated in the singular)
pancreatitis	(păn´´krē-ah-tī´tĭs)	acute or chronic inflammation of the pancreas
peripheral edema	(pĕ-rĭf´ĕr-al ĕ-dē´mah)	abnormally large amounts of fluid within the hands or feet; swollen hands or feet due to this fluid
peritoneal signs	(pĕr´´ĭ-tō-nē´ăl)	indications of disease or abnormality in the peritoneum by touching and listening over the abdominal cavity
protocol		an explicit, detailed plan
Provera®	(prō-vĕr´ah)	trade name for drug used to treat some carcinomas and abnormal uterine bleeding

R

remote appendectomy		removal of the vermiform appendix years ago, perhaps in childhood
retrograde		moving backward or against the usual direction of flow
Rokitansky-Aschoff sinuses	(rō´´kĭ-tăn´skē ăsh´ŏf)	small outpouchings of the mucosa of the gallbladder extending through the muscular layer

| running | | in regard to surgical sutures, the opposite of interrupted sutures; continuous sutures with the stitching fastened at each end by a knot |

S

scapular	(skăp´ū-lăr)	referring to the shoulder blade or the shoulder blade area
segs		acceptable medical jargon; shortened version of segmented neutrophils, which are white blood cells; a part of the differential white blood cell count
sepsis	(sĕp´sĭs)	the presence in the blood or other tissues of toxic organisms
SMA		sequential multiple analyzer; a machine for automated chemical analysis of blood or serum; sometimes dictated as SMA-6 or SMA-12, etc., depending on the number of tests being done on one sample at one time
SOB		shortness of breath
sonogram	(sō´nō-grăm)	a record or display obtained by ultrasonic scanning
stone basket		surgical instrument shaped like a basket and used to retrieve stones from the common bile duct
suspension		a condition of temporary cessation, as of animation, of pain, or of any vital process; urinary bladder suspension refers to a procedure whereby a prolapsed or fallen bladder is surgically tacked back into place

T

| transfixed | | pierced through and through with a sharp instrument |

U

urgency   the sudden compelling urge to urinate

W

waxed and waned   this phase refers to the increase of and
                                                           the subsequent diminishing of an object
                                                           or symptoms; like the moon waxes and
                                                           wanes every month, so may symptoms
                                                           wax and wane

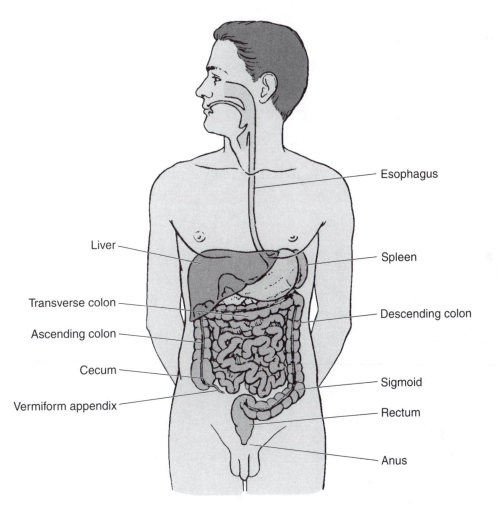

7-1. The digestive system.

Case 8: The Endocrine System

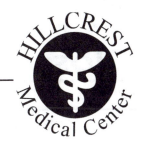

Patient Name

Gerald Edwards

Address

309 North Fifth Street
Miami, FL 33133-4038

Situation

This known diabetic patient had an ulcerated area on one foot. His podiatrist referred the patient to the emergency room at Hillcrest Medical Center. The doctor in the emergency room admitted the patient and requested both the podiatrist and an ophthalmologist to see the patient in consultation. This was done, and the podiatrist performed necessary surgery, submitting the tissue to a pathologist for evaluation and diagnosis. The admitting doctor also ordered an MRI to be done by a radiologist who specializes in nuclear medicine. After all consultations, evaluations, and treatment were completed, the patient was discharged in improved condition. He will be followed by both the podiatrist and the ophthalmologist.

Review Illustration 8-1, Bones of the Foot, on page 134 and Illustration 8-2, The Endocrine System, on page 135.

Student Name _____

Patient: Gerald Edwards

Sequence of Reports	Date Completed	Grade
History and Physical Examination	_____	_____
Request for Consultation x 2	_____	_____
Radiology Report	_____	_____
Operative Report	_____	_____
Pathology Report	_____	_____
Discharge Summary	_____	_____

Enter the date of completion for each report. When you have finished all reports, tear this sheet out, staple it to the front of the reports (in the order listed above), and give the completed reports to your instructor.

Glossary for Case 8
WORDS & PHONETIC PRONUNCIATIONS   DEFINITIONS

A

acute	(ah-kūt´)	having a short and relatively severe course
aerobic	(ā-ĕr-ō´bĭk)	having molecular oxygen present
anaerobic	(ăn´´ā-ĕr-ō´bĭk)	lacking molecular oxygen
Augmentin®	(awg-mĕn´tĭn)	antibiotic (trade name)

B

| bacteriostatic saline | (băk-tē´´ rē-ō-stăt´ĭk sā´lēn) | salt and water solution designed to inhibit the growth or multiplication of bacteria |
| beta streptococci | (bā´tah strĕp´´tō-kŏk´sī) | often dictated "beta strep," this refers to organisms of the genus *Streptococcus* capable of hemolyzing (dissolving) the red blood cell membrane; identified on microbacterial culture media by the clear zone produced around the bacterial colony |

C

calor	(kā´lŏr)	heat
cellulitis	(sĕl´´ū-lī´tĭs)	inflammation of connective tissue
Charcot's disease	(shăr-kōz´)	neuropathic arthropathy (a joint disease)
Cipro®	(sĭ-prō)	antibiotic (trade name)
cuneiform	(kū-nē´ĭ-fŏrm)	shaped like a wedge

D

debridement	(dā-brēd´maw) [Fr.] (dĭ-brēd´mĕnt)	removal of foreign material or contaminated tissue from and/or adjacent to a traumatic or infected lesion
defervesced	(dĕf´´ĕr-vĕsd´)	a reduction of fever
digit	(dĭj´ĭt)	a finger or toe
dorsal	(dŏr´săl)	pertaining to the back
dorsalis [L.]	(dŏr-sā´lĭs)	a term denoting a position closer to the back surface
dorsolateral	(dŏr´´sō-lăt´ĕr-ăl)	pertaining to the back and the side
dot and blot hemorrhages		a pathologic condition; tiny, round hemorrhages in the retina usually associated with diabetes mellitus
D.P.M.		Doctor of Podiatric Medicine

E

edentulous	(ē-dĕn´tū-lŭs)	without teeth
encephalitis	(ĕn´´sĕf-ah-lī´tĭs)	inflammation of the brain
erythematous	(ĕr´´ĭ-thĕm´ah-tŭs)	characterized by erythema (redness of the skin)
eschar	(ĕs´kăr)	a slough produced either by a thermal burn, by a corrosive application, or by gangrene

F

fundus	(fŭn´dŭs)	the bottom or base of anything

G

gallium	(găl´ē-ŭm)	a metal liquid at room temperature; symbol Ga

| glycosylated | (glī-kō´sĭ-lāt´´ĕd) | having formed a linkage with a glycosyl (carbohydrate) group |

H

| hyperkeratotic | (hī´´pĕr-kĕr´´ah-tŏt´ĭk) | excessive development or retention of keratin (protein of skin, hair, and nails) |

I

| I&D | | incision and drainage |

M

macula	(măk´ū-lah)	a stain, spot, or thickening
medial	(mē´dē-ăl)	pertaining to the middle
metatarsal	(mĕt´´ah-tăr´săl)	pertaining to the metatarsus (the part of the foot between the tarsus and the toes)
mm Hg		millimeters of mercury
MRI		magnetic resonance imaging (a radiologic procedure)

N

neovascularization	(nē´´ō-văs´´kū-lăr-ī-zā´shŭn)	new blood vessel formation in either abnormal tissue or in abnormal position
neuropathy	(nū-rŏp´ah-thē)	disease of the peripheral nervous system
NKA (NKDA)		no known allergies (no known drug allergies)
Nu-gauze®	(nū´gawz)	surgical dressing (trade name)

O

| osseous | (ŏs´ē-ŭs) | of the nature or quality of bone; bony |
| osteomyelitis | (ŏs´´tē-ō-mī´´ĕ-lī´tĭs) | inflammation of bone caused by a pyogenic organism |

P

plantar	(plăn´tăr)	pertaining to the sole of the foot

R

retinopathy	(rĕt´´ĭ-nŏp´ah-thē)	disease of the retina

S

sanguinopurulent	(săng´´gwĭ-nō-pū´rū-lĕnt)	containing both blood and pus

T

T&A		tonsils and adenoids, tonsillectomy and adenoidectomy
tabes dorsalis [L.]	(tā´bēz dŏr-sā´lĭs)	a degeneration of the dorsal column of the spinal cord and of the sensory nerve trunks
tarsal	(tahr´săl)	pertaining to the instep; any of the seven bones of the tarsus
tendinous	(tĕn´dĭ-nŭs)	pertaining to a tendon
tie-over dressing		a dressing placed over a skin graft and tied on by sutures that have been left long enough for that purpose
Trental®	(trĕn´tăl)	a drug used to treat peripheral vascular disease (trade name)
tympanic	(tĭm-păn´ĭk)	pertaining to the tympanic membrane that separates the middle from the external ear

U

Unasyn®	(ū´nă-sĭn)	antibiotic (trade name)

V

venous	(vē´nŭs)	pertaining to a vein or veins
vitreous	(vĭt´rē-ŭs)	glasslike

W

| Webril® padding | (wĕb´rĭl) | material used during surgery to protect the skin of the extremity under a tourniquet (trade name) |

X

| Xeroflo® | (zē´rō-flō) | gauze dressing (trade name) |

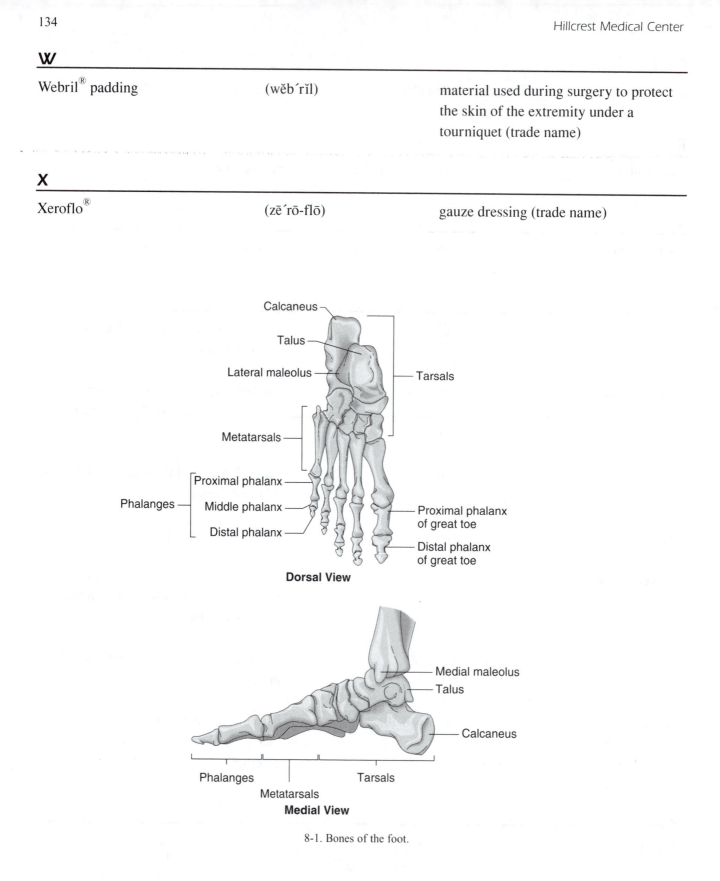

8-1. Bones of the foot.

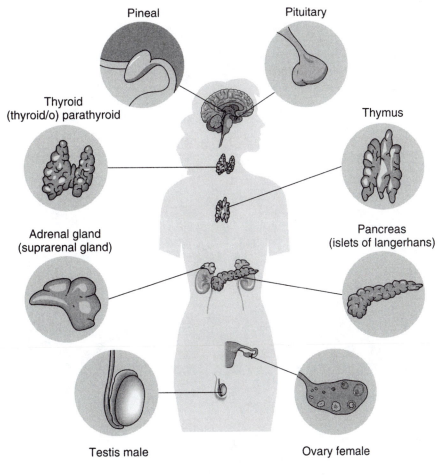

Pineal

Pituitary

Thyroid
(thyroid/o) parathyroid

Thymus

Adrenal gland
(suprarenal gland)

Pancreas
(islets of langerhans)

Testis male

Ovary female

8-2. The endocrine system.

Case 9: The Lymphatic System

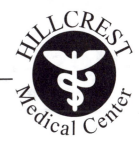

Patient Name

Mark Thomas

Address

9038 S.W. 45th Terrace
South Miami, FL 33165-5912

Situation

This young man had been suffering from shortness of breath and, with his history of lymphoma, finally went to see a physician, a surgeon, who admitted him to Hillcrest. In the subsequent work-up the patient's oncologist was notified of the readmission, and radiology was involved in a special study. After the planned surgical procedure the tissue removed was submitted to pathology for evaluation. On discharge the patient's shortness of breath was improved, and he was scheduled to go back on chemotherapy and have a GI work-up as an outpatient.

Review Illustration 9-1, The Lymphatic System, on page 143.

Student Name _____

Patient: Mark Thomas

Sequence of Reports	Date Completed	Grade
History and Physical Examination	_____	_____
Operative Report	_____	_____
Pathology Report	_____	_____
Radiology Report	_____	_____
Discharge Summary	_____	_____

Enter the date of completion for each report. When you have finished all reports, tear this sheet out, staple it to the front of the reports (in the order listed above), and give the completed reports to your instructor.

Glossary for Case 9

WORDS & PHONETIC PRONUNCIATIONS   DEFINITIONS

A

abdominal	(ăb-dŏm´ĭ-năl)	pertaining to the abdomen
Adriamycin®	(ā´´drē-ah-mī´sĭn)	antibiotic used only in chemotherapy (trade name)
amiodarone	(ah-mē´ō-dah-rŏn´´)	antiarrhythmic drug (generic)
anergy panel	(ăn´ĕr-jē)	a group of substances to which a patient's allergic susceptibility is tested
apex	(a´pĕks)	a general term used to designate the top of a body, organ, or part
arrhythmia	(ah-rĭth´mē-ah)	any variation from the normal rhythm of the heartbeat
arteriole	(ăr-tē´rē-ōl)	a minute arterial branch
atraumatic	(ā´´traw-măt´ĭk)	not inflicting or causing damage or injury; not damaged or injured
atropine	(ăt´rō-pēn)	generic drug used preoperatively as a muscle relaxer and to inhibit salivation and secretions; it has other uses, too
axilla	(ăk-sĭl´ah)	armpit (pl. axillae)

B

bibasilar rales	(bī´băs´ĭ-lăr rahls)	crackling sounds heard in the bases of both lungs
bronchomalacia	(brŏng´´kō-mah-lā´shē-ah)	degeneration of elastic and connective tissue of bronchi and trachea
bronchoscope	(brŏng´kō-skōp)	instrument with which to examine the bronchi

| bronchoscopy | (brŏng-kŏs´kō-pē) | examination of the bronchi through a bronchoscope |
| bronchospasm | (brŏng´kō-spăzm) | spasmodic contraction of the smooth muscle of the bronchi |

C

cardiac	(kăr´dē-ăk)	pertaining to the heart
carina	(kah-rī´nah)	a ridgelike structure
costophrenic	(kŏs´´tō-frĕn´ĭk)	pertaining to the ribs and diaphragm
cytology	(sī-tŏl´ō-jē)	the study of cells

D

diabetes mellitus	(dī´´ah-bē´tēz mĕ-lī´tŭs) (dī´´ah-bē´tēz mĕl´lĭ-tŭs)	a metabolic disease due to an abnormality of insulin; diabetes is associated with multiple complications of various organs and systems
DLCO		diffusing capacity of the lung for carbon monoxide
dorsalis pedis [L.]	(dor-sā´lĭs pē´dĭs)	a term denoting a position closer to the back surface of the foot

E

Ecotrin®	(ĕk´ō-trĭn)	nonsteroidal anti-inflammatory drug (trade name)
endobronchial	(ĕn´´dō-brŏng´kē-ăl)	pertaining to within the bronchi
epigastric	(ĕp´´ĭ-găs´trĭk)	pertaining to the epigastrium
epigastrium	(ĕp´´ĭ-găs´trē-ŭm)	the upper middle region of the abdomen
esophageal reflux	(ĕ-sŏf´´ah-jē´ăl rē´flŭks)	a backward flow or regurgitation of stomach

F

FEV$_1$		forced expiratory volume in one second (part of the pulmonary function tests)
FVC		forced vital capacity (part of the pulmonary function tests)

G

gait	(gāt)	the manner or style of walking
gastritis	(găs-trī´tĭs)	inflammation of the stomach

H

heaves	(hēvz)	a respiratory disturbance characterized by partially forced expiration
hematochezia	(hēm´´ah-tō-kē´zē-ah)	the passage of bloody stools
Hemoccult®	(hē´mō-kŭlt)	trade name for a test used to detect hidden blood, usually in stool ("Hem negative" may be dictated)
hilar	(hī´lăr)	pertaining to a hilus (depression at that part of an organ where the vessels and nerves enter)
holosystolic murmur	(hŏl´´ō-sĭs-tŏl´ĭk mŭr´mŭr)	heart sound heard over the entire systole, or the period of contraction; also called pansystolic murmur
HTN		hypertension
hypokinesis	(hī´´pō-kī-nē´sĭs)	abnormally decreased mobility

I

IM		intramuscularly; within the muscle(s)
infrahilar	(ĭn´´frah-hī´lăr)	below the hilum (a depression or pit)

J

jugulovenous	(jŭg´´ū-lō-vē´nŭs)	referring to the jugular vein in the neck

L

Lasix®	(lā´sĭks)	trade name for a drug used to manage edema and/or hypertension
lavage	(lah-vahzh´)	irrigation of an organ
LVEF		left ventricular ejection fraction (a cardiac term)

M

macrophage	(măk´rō-fāj)	large red blood cells with a round or indented nucleus
morphine	(mōr´fēn)	generic drug used as a narcotic; pain medication
MUGA		multiple gated acquisition (scan), a radiologic procedure

N

naris	(nā´rĭs)	one of the openings of the nasal cavity; a nostril (pl. nares)
nebulizer	(nĕb´ū-līz´´ĕr)	an atomizer; a device for throwing a spray
necrosis	(nĕ-krō´sĭs)	cell death
non-Hodgkin's lymphoma	(lĭm-fō´mah)	a group of malignant lymphomas; a neoplasm arising from the lymphatics; the most common manifestation is the painless enlargement of one or more lymph nodes

O

oximetry	(ŏk-sĭm´ē-trē)	determination of the oxygen saturation of arterial blood using an oximeter (instrument)

P

Pepcid®	(pĕp´sĭd)	blocker drug to heal ulcers (trade name)

PFT		pulmonary function test
pneumothorax	(nū´´mō-thō´răks)	an accumulation of air or gas in the pleural space
PPD		purified protein derivative (of tuberculin); skin test for tuberculosis
Propacet®	(prō´pă-sĕt)	trade name for a pain medication

R

RDW		red (cell) distribution width (a lab term)

S

S/P		status post; used to indicate the patient's condition after a procedure, i.e., status post appendectomy or status post chemotherapy
sternal	(stĕr´năl)	pertaining to the sternum

T

Tenormin®	(tĕn´ŏr-mĭn)	trade name of drug used to treat angina and hypertension; also used for migraine headaches
thrill	(thrĭl)	a sensation or vibration felt by the examiner on palpation of the body (often a cardiac term)
transbronchial	(trăns-brŏng´kē-ăl)	referring to across the bronchus sideways

V

Vasotec®	(vā´zō-tĕk)	inhibitor drug used for hypertension (trade name)
Ventolin®	(vĕn´tō-lĭn)	trade name for a drug used in asthma and other respiratory diseases to reverse airway obstruction

Versed®	(vĕr-sĕd´)	a nonbarbiturate agent given intravenously either preoperatively or during surgery to produce both sedation and amnesia
VP-16		a chemotherapy drug administered intravenously; trade name is VePesid®

Cervical nodes

Left subclavian vein
(a lymph-related blood vessel)

Axillary nodes

Thoracic duct

Mammary plexus

Right lymphatic duct

Cubital nodes

Iliac nodes

Inguinal nodes

Popliteal nodes

9-1. The lymphatic system.

Case 10: The Respiratory System

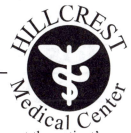

Patient Name

Scott Chandler

Address

14302 Briarbend
Key Biscayne, FL 33149-6747

Situation

This elderly patient found himself in respiratory distress and was brought by ambulance to Hillcrest emergency room early one morning. The emergency room physicians together with a pulmonary/thoracic surgeon performed emergency surgery. The radiology department did serial chest x-rays to determine whether or not the patient's lung remained expanded. Due to a worsening in the patient's respiratory status, the surgeon performed a second procedure, and radiology continued to keep a close check on his chest and lungs. After continued complications and significant deterioration in the patient's condition, the pulmonary/thoracic surgeon was requested to assess the patient. He recommended transfer to the larger facility at Forrest General Medical Center for more complicated surgery. The patient was therefore transferred to Forrest General for further evaluation and care by the consultant.

Review Illustration 10-1, The Respiratory System, on page 150

Student Name _____

Patient: Scott Chandler

Sequence of Reports	Date Completed	Grade
History and Physical Examination	_____	_____
Operative Report No. 1	_____	_____
Radiology Report x 2	_____	_____
Operative Report No. 2	_____	_____
Radiology Report	_____	_____
Request for Consultation	_____	_____
Discharge Summary	_____	_____

Enter the date of completion for each report. When you have finished all reports, tear this sheet out, staple it to the front of the reports (in the order listed above), and give the completed reports to your instructor.

Glossary for Case 10
WORDS & PHONETIC PRONUNCIATIONS   DEFINITIONS

A

ablation	(ăb-lā´shŭn)	separation or detachment; removal of a part, especially by cutting
anesthetize	(ah-nĕs´thĕ-tīz)	to put under the influence of anesthetics—drugs or agents used to abolish the sensation of pain
aorta	(ā-ŏr´tah)	the main trunk of the arterial system, conveying blood from the heart

B

benzoin	(bĕn´zoin)	a topical antiseptic, generic
bronchodilator	(brŏng´´kō-dī-lā´tŏr)	dilating or expanding the air passages of the lungs
bronchopleural	(brŏng´´kō-ploor´ăl)	pertaining to a bronchus and the pleura

C

cannula	(kăn´ū-lah)	a tube for insertion into a duct or cavity
catheter	(kăth´ĕ-tĕr)	a tubular, flexible surgical instrument for either withdrawing fluids from or introducing fluids into a cavity of the body
ciprofloxin	(sĭp´´rō-flŏx´ĭn)	generic name for a broad-spectrum antibiotic
COPD		chronic obstructive pulmonary disease

D

decubitus	(dē-kū´bĭ-tŭs)	the position assumed in lying down (decubitus position, decubitus ulcers)

E

| emergent | (ē-mĕr´jĕnt) | pertaining to an emergency |

| emphysema | (ĕm´´fĭ-sē´mah) | a pathologic accumulation of air in tissues or organs—applied especially to such a condition of the lungs |

F

| fistula | (fĭs´tū-lah) | an abnormal passage, usually between two internal organs or leading from an internal organ to the surface of the body |

H

| hemithorax | (hēm´´ē-thō´răks) | one side of the chest |

| hemostat | (hē´mō-stăt) | a small surgical clamp for constricting a blood vessel |

| HJR | | hepatojugular reflux (a GI term) |

| hypertension | (hī´´pĕr-tĕn´shŭn) | persistently high arterial blood pressure |

I

| ichthyosis | (ĭk´´thē-ō´sĭs) | dryness and fish-like scaling of the skin |

L

| loculate | (lŏk´ū-lāt) | divided into loculi (cavities) |

| loculus | (lŏk´ū-lŭs) | a small space or cavity (pl. loculi) |

M

| marked | | noticeable; to an extreme |

P

| PCO_2 | | partial pressure (or tension) of carbon dioxide (done on blood gas studies) |

| percutaneous | (pĕr´´kū-tā´nē-ŭs) | performed through the skin |

pH		hydrogen ion concentration in urine, blood, and other body fluids (neutral = 7.00; more than 7.00 is alkaline; less than 7.00 is acidic). NOTE; Always pH, even at beginning of sentence.
pleural vac	(ploor´ăl văk)	thoracic drainage system (equipment)
pleurodesis	(ploo-rō-dē´sĭs)	the production of adhesions between the parietal and the visceral pleura
PO$_2$		partial pressure (tension) of oxygen (a blood gas term)
portable chest		medical jargon pertaining to the equipment used and the process of obtaining a chest x-ray outside of the radiology department
Proventil®	(prō-věn´tĭl)	bronchodilator (trade name)
Pseudomonas aeruginosa	(soo´´dō-mō´năs ě´´rū-gĭn-ō´sah)	the type of bacterial species of the genus, and the only one pathogenic for man, made up of microorganisms that produce the blue-green pigment that gives the color to "blue pus" observed in certain suppurative infections
pulmonary	(pŭl´mō-něr´´ē)	pertaining to the lungs

R

radiograph	(rā´dē-o-grăf´´)	x-ray
resolution		the subsidence of a pathologic state, as the subsidence of an inflammation or the softening and disappearance of a swelling
Rocephin®	(rō-sěf´ĭn)	antibiotic (trade name)

S

sclerotherapy	(sklĕ´´rō-thĕr´ah-pē)	treatment involving the injection of a sclerosing or hardening solution into vessels or tissues
stat	(stăt)	abbreviation for [L.] statim (immediately); largely misused, it is meant to convey a life or death emergency
Streptococcus	(strĕp´´tō-kŏk´ŭs)	bacteria growing in chains found in human mouth and intestine; sometimes they cause disease
subcutaneous	(sŭb´´kū-ta-nē-ŭs)	beneath the skin
subtherapeutic	(sŭb´´thĕr´ah-pū´tĭk)	a less than therapeutic level, usually referring to the blood level of a particular drug or medication

T

tachycardia	(tăk´´ē-kăr´dē-ah)	excessive rapidity in the action of the heart
Theo-Dur®	(thē´ō-dŭr)	trade name for theophylline, a bronchodilator used in patients with asthma or COPD
theophylline	(thē-ŏf´ĭ-lĭn)	a smooth muscle relaxant, used chiefly for its bronchodilator effect
thoracic	(thō-răs´ĭk)	pertaining to the chest
thoracostomy	(thō´´rah-kŏs´tō-mē)	surgical creation of an opening in the wall of the chest for the purpose of drainage
thoracotomy	(thō´´rah-kŏt´ō-mē)	surgical incision of the wall of the chest

X

Xylocaine®	(zī´lō-kān)	trade name for preparations of lidocaine

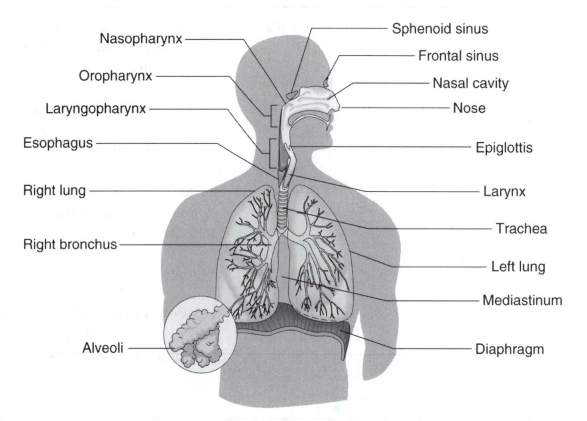

Nasopharynx

Oropharynx

Laryngopharynx

Esophagus

Right lung

Right bronchus

Alveoli

Sphenoid sinus

Frontal sinus

Nasal cavity

Nose

Epiglottis

Larynx

Trachea

Left lung

Mediastinum

Diaphragm

10-1. The respiratory system.

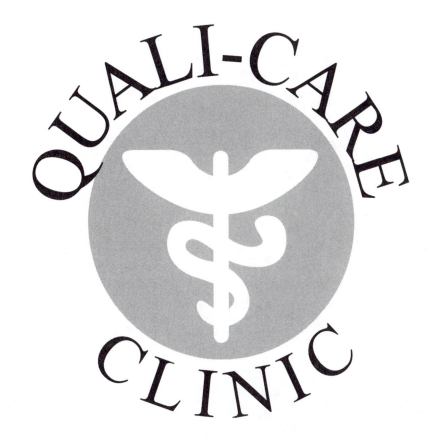

Welcome to Quali-Care Clinic

You will be transcribing outpatient medical reports for Quali-Care Clinic, a medical facility housed in a freestanding office building adjacent to Hillcrest Medical Center and containing the offices of physicians and health care providers from 12 different medical specialties. Those in the specialties of Family Practice and Internal Medicine act as primary care physicians (PCPs) who see their patients on a regular basis, paying close attention to their overall well-being, and referring them to specialists or Hillcrest Medical Center for further evaluation and treatment as necessary. (NOTE: PCPs for female patients include Gynecology and Obstetrics.)

You will be transcribing 20 outpatient reports that relate to these medical specialty areas. These reports demonstrate variations in style, format, and content common to the dictating habits of the originators of medical records—habits usually learned while in medical school. Model Report Form 9 (page 36) shows a model HPIP report (history, physical, impression, plan) and Model Report Form 10 (page 37) shows a model SOAP report (subjective, objective, assessment, plan). These two formats or variations thereof are the mainstay of the physicians' outpatient medical record (chart) on each patient. The SOAP format is less formal and generally used in doctors' chart notes. Variations in this format are less likely than in the HPIP; however, each physician personalizes a format using a preferred style.

Included in a medical record would also be patient demographic information, the next of kin, what to do in case of emergency, laboratory and x-ray results, vital signs written in at each visit, chart notes by the physician, etc. The doctor may dictate chart notes after each patient visit and telephone call *or* these notes may be handwritten. Elderly or very ill patients or families may be counseled regarding a living will, a directive to physicians, or otherwise asked to indicate their wishes should a terminal situation exist. This may be referred to as "DNR" status or a "no code" status, which means do not resuscitate (DNR) should cardiac or respiratory failure occur, and do not allow hospital or emergency personnel to institute lifesaving measures (like a "Code Blue"). There are many variations in this type of planning, but patients and their families have the right and the responsibility to state their wishes and to have them honored.

When a patient is referred to a specialist, any number of special examinations or procedures, both invasive and noninvasive, may occur. If all attempts to cure a patient fail using outpatient measures, then inpatient measures must follow. This involves admission to a hospital, either Hillcrest, the adjacent 400-bed medical center, or Forrest General, the larger, teaching hospital that includes a major trauma center, organ transplant facility, burn center, and rehabilitation unit.

In summary, outpatient care is done on the following levels:

1. Telephone calls to the PCP
2. Scheduled appointments with the PCP
3. Requests for lab and x-rays for diagnostic purposes
4. Referral to a specialist (or consultant) for further evaluation and treatment
5. Treatment in the specialist's (or consultant's) office with more advanced, noninvasive procedures
6. Invasive procedures that include surgery
7. Transfer to Hillcrest Medical Center for further evaluation and treatment
8. Transfer to Forrest General Hospital, if necessary
9. Aftercare to include physical therapy, occupational therapy, nursing home care—either skilled (short-term) or custodial (long-term)—with appropriate follow-up by the original PCP

Extensive records are kept at each level of patient care, and this involves dictation and transcription. Remember, *legally*, what was not written down or transcribed was not done. MTs create records that are vital to patient care and are legal documents subject to subpoena. They also create a medical history that is the basis for reimbursement from third-party payers (insurance companies) and for research purposes.

We hope that transcribing the outpatient reports proves to be a valuable learning experience.

Sincerely,

Allison Poole

Allison Poole, CMT, RRA
Director, Medical Records Department

QUALI-CARE CLINIC OUTPATIENT REPORTS LOG

Student Name _____

Enter the date of completion for each Quali-Care Clinic outpatient report in the following log. When you have finished all of the reports, tear this sheet out, staple it to the front of the reports, and give the completed reports to your instructor. Or, adapt this log as needed for your own use.

Report # & Patient Name	Date Completed	Grade
Report 1: Doris Moore		
Report 2: Wes Olston		
Report 3: Alice Montfort		
Report 4: Winnie Cooper		
Report 5: Letty Brown		
Report 6: Howard Huff		
Report 7: Linda Brody		
Report 8: Melinda Klein		
Report 9: Adele Aguilar		
Report 10: Bess Martin		
Report 11: Carol White		
Report 12: Nicolle Brooks		
Report 13: Lynda Shoemaker		
Report 14: John J. Wagner		
Report 15: Barbara Ann Richards		
Report 16: Jim Wilson		
Report 17: Joseph Patrick		
Report 18: George Nandor		
Report 19: Leslie Arispe		
Report 20: B. Christine Anello		

OUTPATIENT REPORTS

This section contains a brief explanation of each patient's reason for receiving outpatient medical care along with a glossary of medical terms found in each report.

Report 1: Doris Moore is a dialysis patient due to diabetic-associated kidney failure. She has developed an infection in her left leg at her graft site, and her PCP, Dr. Lewis, has sent her to radiology for a CT scan of that leg to get a definitive diagnosis. See Hemodialysis Illustration on page 156.

Words & Phonetic Pronunciations
Definitions

arteriosclerosis	(ahr-tēr´´ē-ō-sklĕ-rō´sĭs)	thickening and loss of elasticity (hardening) of arterial walls
CT scan		computed tomography scan (radiology procedure)
hematoma	(hē´´mah-tō´mah)	a localized collection of blood, usually clotted, in an organ, space, or tissue, due to a break in the wall of a blood vessel
hemodialysis site	(hē´´mō-dī-ăl´ĭ-sĭs)	the site where the removal of certain elements from the blood by means of a hemodialyzer is done
midinferior	(mĭd-ĭn-fēr´ē-ŏr)	in the middle and directed downward
multiple axial images		many pictures taken by rotating around the axis of the body
retroperitoneum	(rĕt´´rō-pĕr´´ĭ-tō-nē´ŭm)	the retroperitoneal space (behind the peritoneum)

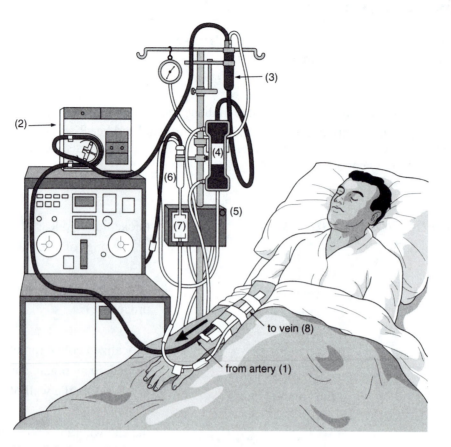

Hemodialysis. (1) Blood leaves the body via an artery. (2) Arterial blood passes through the blood pump. (3) Blood is filtered to remove any clots. (4) Blood passes through the dialyzer. (5) Blood passes into the venous blood line. (6) Blood is filtered to remove any clots. (7) Blood flows through the air detector. (8) Blood returns to the client through the venous blood line.

Report 2: Wes Olston was sent to an orthopedist in consultation because of a pelvic fracture suffered in a car accident. See Patient History Form on page 158.

Words & Phonetic Pronunciations   ## Definitions

ambulation	(ăm´´bū-lā´shŭn)	the act of walking
antalgic gait	(ăn-tăl´gĭk gāt)	the manner of walking when there is pain on weight-bearing
AP		anteroposterior (a direction)
pubic rami	(pū´bĭk rā´mī)	a branch of the hip bone (ramus, sing.)

PATIENT HISTORY FORM

Patient Name:_____ Date _____

	DOCTOR/THERAPIST USE ONLY

1. PLEASE CHECK THE AREA OF YOUR <u>MAJOR</u> COMPLAINT:
   - ☐ HEADACHE ☐ NECK ☐ BETWEEN SHOULDERS ☐ LOW BACK
   - ☐ SHOULDER ☐ HIP ☐ ARM ☐ LEG
2. HOW DID THIS EPISODE BEGIN (CHECK APPROPRIATE ANSWER)?
   - ☐ LIFTING ☐ HIT IN BACK
   - ☐ TWISTING ☐ AUTO ACCIDENT → DATE OF INJURY:_____
   - ☐ PUSHING ☐ ON THE JOB → DATE OF INJURY:_____
   - ☐ PULLING ☐ UNKNOWN
   - ☐ BENDING ☐ OTHER: _____
     _____
3. WHEN DID THIS EPISODE OF PAIN BEGIN?_____
4. HAVE YOU HAD A SIMILAR EPISODE BEFORE? ☐ YES ☐ NO
5. WHAT TESTS HAVE YOU HAD AND WHAT ARE THE RESULTS?
   1.
   2.
   3.
   4.
6. LIST DOCTORS & THERAPISTS YOU HAVE SEEN & THE RESULTS.
   1.
   2.
   3.
   4.
7. WHAT HAVE YOU BEEN TOLD IS WRONG?
   - ☐ PINCHED NERVE ☐ ARTHRITIS
   - ☐ SLIPPED DISC ☐ NOT TOLD
   - ☐ PULLED MUSCLE
   - ☐ OTHER: _____
8. FOR YOUR NECK OR BACK, HAVE YOU EVER HAD:
   - ☐ HOSPITALIZATION ☐ BONE SCAN
   - ☐ X-RAYS ☐ MYELOGRAM
   - ☐ CAT SCAN ☐ EMG
   - ☐ MRI SCAN ☐ NONE
   - ☐ OTHER: _____
9. HAVE YOU TAKEN ANY MEDICINE FOR THIS PROBLEM?
   - ☐ NONE ☐ FELDENE ☐ IBUPROFEN
   - ☐ MOTRIN ☐ MECLOMEN ☐ ALEVE
   - ☐ NALFON ☐ ORUDIS ☐ ASPIRIN
   - ☐ NAPROSYN ☐ ORUVAIL ☐ TYLENOL
   - ☐ CLINORIL ☐ RELAFEN ☐ CORTISONE: STEROIDS
   - ☐ INDOCIN ☐ LODINE   PREDNISONE
   - ☐ TOLECTIN ☐ ADVIL   DECADRON
   - ☐ OTHER: _____   MEDROL

10. HAVE YOU HAD:

	YES	NO	BETTER	WORSE	SAME
PHYSICAL THERAPY	☐	☐	☐	☐	☐
CORSET OR BRACE	☐	☐	☐	☐	☐
CHIROPRACTIC	☐	☐	☐	☐	☐
MASSAGE	☐	☐	☐	☐	☐
BACK SURGERY	☐	☐	☐	☐	☐
ACUPUNCTURE	☐	☐	☐	☐	☐
CORTISONE SHOT	☐	☐	☐	☐	☐

Patient Name:_____

11. USE THESE SYMBOLS TO SHOW AREA ON THE DRAWINGS WHERE YOU HAVE SYMPTOMS:

>>>ACHE ☐ ☐ NUMBNESS ☐ ☐ PINS & NEEDLES X X BURNING //// STABBING

12. ARE YOUR SYMPTOMS GETTING: ☐ BETTER ☐ SAME ☐ WORSE

13. PLEASE CHECK ONE ANSWER IF IT APPLIES TO YOU:
   ☐ BACK (NECK) PAIN IS WORSE THAN LEG (ARM) PAIN
   ☐ BACK (NECK) PAIN EQUALS LEG (ARM) PAIN
   ☐ LEG (ARM) PAIN IS WORSE THAN BACK (NECK) PAIN

14. PLEASE CHECK ALL OF THE FOLLOWING THAT BEST DESCRIBE YOUR PAIN:
   ☐ CONSTANT   ☐ WAKES YOU UP AT NIGHT
   ☐ DAILY   ☐ WORSE WITH COUGH/SNEEZE
   ☐ WORSE IN MORNING   ☐ WORSE WITH ACTIVITY

15. CHECK THE APPROPRIATE BOXES REGARDING YOUR PAIN:

	WORSE	BETTER	NO CHANGE
SITTING	☐	☐	☐
STANDING	☐	☐	☐
GETTING UP FROM SITTING	☐	☐	☐
BENDING FORWARD	☐	☐	☐
LEANING BACKWARD	☐	☐	☐
LIFTING	☐	☐	☐
WALKING	☐	☐	☐
REST	☐	☐	☐
LYING ON BACK	☐	☐	☐
LYING ON STOMACH	☐	☐	☐
MENSTRUAL PERIODS	☐	☐	☐

16. HAVE YOU LOST CONTROL OF YOUR BOWELS OR BLADDER?
   ☐ YES   ☐ NO

DOCTOR/THERAPIST USE ONLY

Report 3: Alice Montfort is undergoing a complicated pregnancy and was sent by her PCP, Dr. Rumen, to a neurologist for an EEG to evaluate her headaches.

Words & Phonetic Pronunciations

Definitions

asymmetry	(ă-sĭm´ĕ-trē)	dissimilarity in the corresponding parts or organs on opposite sides of the body that are normally alike
EEG		electroencephalogram
epileptiform	(ĕp´´ĭ-lĕp´tĭ-fŏrm)	resembling epilepsy or its manifestations
hypertension	(hī´´pĕr-tĕn´shŭn)	high arterial blood pressure
posterior	(pŏs-tēr´ē-ŏr)	situated in back of, or in the back part of, or affecting the back part of a structure

Report 4: Winnie Cooper has had trouble swallowing for some time. She has been sent by her PCP, Dr. Farinacci, to a gastroenterologist for a work-up.

Words & Phonetic Pronunciations

Definitions

bolus	(bō´lŭs)	a rounded mass of food
dyspepsia	(dĭs-pĕp´sē-ah)	impairment of the power or function of digestion
dysphagia	(dĭs-fā´jē-ah)	difficulty in swallowing
esophageal	(ĕ-sŏf´´ah-jē´ăl)	pertaining to the esophagus (the musculomembranous passage extending from the pharynx to the stomach)
GI endoscopy	(ĕn-dŏs´kō-pē)	visual inspection of the gastrointestinal tract by means of an endoscope
hematochezia	(hĕm´´ah-tō-kē´zē-ah)	the passage of bloody stools
Hemoccult®	(hē´mō-kŭlt)	trade name for a test used to detect hidden blood, usually in stool
reflux	(rē´flŭks)	a backward or return flow
substernal	(sŭb-stĕr´năl)	situated beneath or inferior to the sternum
symptomatology	(sĭmp´´tō-mah-tŏl´ō-jē)	the combined symptoms of a disease

Report 5: Letty Brown is a young woman with severe itching, who has been sent to a dermatologist for a consultation.

Words & Phonetic Pronunciations

Definitions

Atarax®	(ăt´ah-răks)	trade name for hydroxyzine hydrochloride, antianxiety drug given for severe itching
dermographism	(děr´´mō-grăf´ ĭz-ŭm)	urticaria (hives) due to physical allergy
erythema	(ěr´´ ĭ-thē´mah)	redness of the skin produced by congestion of the capillaries
pruritus	(proo-rī´tŭs)	itching
urticaria	(ŭr´´tĭ-kā´rē-ah)	a vascular reaction (hives) involving the upper dermis
xerosis	(zēr-ō´sĭs)	abnormal dryness, as of the eye, skin, or mouth
xerotic dermatitis	(zēr-ŏt´ĭk děr´´mah-tī´tĭs)	inflammation of dry skin

Report 6: Howard Huff, a dialysis patient due to kidney disease, is having complications. He comes
to his PCP's office for a check-up.

Words & Phonetic Pronunciations

Definitions

| amoxicillin | (ah-mŏks´´ĭ-sĭl´ĭn) | penicillin-type antibiotic |

| Buprenex® | (bū´prĕ-nĕks) | trade name for buprenorphine hydrochloride, a narcotic pain medication |

| biotin | (bī´ō-tĭn) | part of the vitamin B complex, biotin aids in amino acid and fatty acid metabolism |

| captopril | (kăp´tō-prĭl) | an enzyme inhibitor used in the treatment of hypertension and congestive heart failure |

| cellulitis | (sĕl´´ū-lī´tĭs) | an acute, diffuse, spreading, edematous, suppurative inflammation of the deep subcutaneous tissues |

| cephalexin | (sĕf´´ah-lĕk´sĭn) | used in the treatment of infections of the urinary and respiratory tracts and of skin and soft tissue due to sensitive pathogens |

| chlorhexidine | (klŏr-hĕks´ĭ-dēn) | an antibacterial, effective against a wide variety of gram-negative and gram-positive organisms |

| Effexor® | (ē´fĕx-ŏr) | trade name for venlafaxine hydrochloride, an antidepressant medication |

| glomerulonephritis | (glō-mĕr´´ū-lō-nĕ-frī´tĭs) | nephritis accompanied by inflammation of the capillary loops in the glomeruli of the kidney |

| indurated | (ĭn´dū-rāt´´ĕd) | hardened |

| lymphedema | (lĭm´´fĕ-dē´mah) | chronic unilateral or bilateral edema of the extremities due to accumulation of interstitial fluid |

| nares | (nā´rēz) | nostrils |

Nephrox®	(nĕ´frŏx)	trade name for aluminum hydroxide, a drug used to treat hyperacidity (too much acid) or too much phosphate
oxacillin	(ŏk˝ sah-sĭl´ĭn)	penicillin-type antibiotic
PhosLo®	(fŏs´lō)	trade name for calcium acetate, a drug used in end-stage renal failure
staphylococcal skin lesions	(stăf˝´ĭ-lō-kŏk´ăl)	skin lesions caused by the bacteria staphylococcus (sometimes called staph)
urticarial	(ŭr˝´tĭ-kā´rē-ăl)	pertaining to a vascular reaction, usually transient, involving the upper dermis, representing localized edema caused by dilatation and increased permeability of the capillaries, and marked by the development of wheals
vancomycin	(văn˝´kō-mī´sĭn)	antibiotic medication
Xanax®	(zăn´ăks)	trade name for alprazolam, an antianxiety drug
Zantac®	(zăn´tăk)	trade name for ranitidine hydrochloride, a drug used to heal ulcers

Report 7: Linda Brody has the symptoms of a urinary tract infection. Because of a history of urinary tract infections, her PCP has sent her to a urologist for a check-up.

Words & Phonetic Pronunciations

Definitions

costovertebral	(kŏs˝tō-vĕr´tĕ-brăl) (kŏs˝tō-vĕr-tē´brăl)	pertaining to a rib and a vertebra
cystitis	(sĭs-tī´tĭs)	inflammation of the urinary bladder
esterase	(ĕs´tĕr-ās)	an enzyme
Macrobid®	(măk´rō-bĭd)	trade name for nitrofurantoin, an antibiotic used to treat urinary tract infections, miscellaneous antibiotic
NKDA		no known drug allergies
p.o.		(per os) [L.] by mouth
postpartum	(pōst-păr´tŭm)	occurring after childbirth, or after delivery, with reference to the mother
Pyridium®	(pĭ-rĭd´ē-ŭm)	trade name for phenazopyridine hydrochloride, a urinary tract analgesic

Report 8: Melinda Klein was sent to a rheumatologist in consultation because of some musculoskeletal problems with her shoulder. See Illustration on page 167.

Words & Phonetic Pronunciations

Definitions

Aristocort®	(ah-rĭs´tō-cŏrt)	trade name for triamcinolone, a topical and oral corticosteroid anti-inflammatory drug
bursitis	(bĕr-sī´tĭs)	inflammation of a bursa
CBC		complete blood count (a lab test)
densitometer	(dĕn´´sĭ-tŏm´ĕ-tĕr)	an apparatus for determining the density of a liquid
ecchymoses	(ĕk´´ĭ-mo´sēs)	small spots on the skin or mucous membranes forming nonelevated, rounded or irregular, blue or purplish patches
fibromyalgia	(fī´´brō-mī-ăl´jē-ah)	pain in muscle fibers
lidocaine	(lī´dō-kān)	topical anesthetic
lipomatous	(lĭ-pō´mah-tŭs)	pertaining to a benign, soft, rubbery, encapsulated tumor of adipose tissue, usually composed of mature fat cells
osteoporosis	(ŏs´´tē-ō-pō-rō´sĭs)	reduction in the amount of bone mass, leading to fractures after minimal trauma
polymyalgia rheumatica	(pŏl´´ē-mī-ăl´jē-ah roo-măt´ĭ-ka)	pain affecting several muscles due to rheumatism
prednisone	(prĕd´nĭ-sōn)	oral corticosteroid anti-inflammatory drug
PT		prothrombin time, a lab test sometimes dictated "pro time"
PTT		partial thromboplastin time; one test to determine how fast the blood clots

rheumatology (roo´´mah-tŏl´ō-jē) the branch of medicine dealing with rheumatic disorders, their causes, pathology, diagnosis, and treatment

subacromial (sŭb´´ah-krō´mē-ăl) situated below or beneath the acromion (the lateral extension of the spine of the scapula, projecting over the shoulder joint and forming the highest point of the shoulder)

synovitis (sīn´´ō-vī´tĭs) inflammation of a synovial membrane

WNL within normal limits

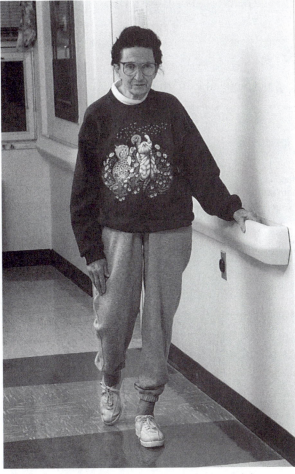

Changes in the bones of the vertebral column result in postural changes.

Report 9: Adele Aguilar is a cancer patient who is having some skin problems while receiving chemotherapy. Because of her serious condition, she is sent to a dermatologist for consultation. See Illustration of pemphigus vulgaris sites below.

Words & Phonetic Pronunciations   ## Definitions

cachectic	(kă-kĕk´tĭk)	pertaining to or characterized by cachexia (general ill health)
hyperpigmented	(hī´´pĕr-pĭg´mĕnt-ĕd)	abnormally increased pigmentation
immunosuppression	(ĭm´´ū-nō-sŭ-prĕsh´ŭn)	the prevention or diminution of the immune response
metastasis	(mĕ-tăs´tah-sĭs)	the transfer of disease from one organ or part to another not directly connected with it (pl. metastases)
pemphigus vulgaris	(pĕm´fĭ-gŭs vŭl-gā´rĭs)	the most common and severe form of pemphigus (a group of chronic, relapsing, sometimes fatal skin diseases)
pleural effusions	(ploor´ăl ĕ-fū´zhŭns)	the escape of fluid into the pleura (the serous membrane investing the lungs and lining the thoracic cavity)

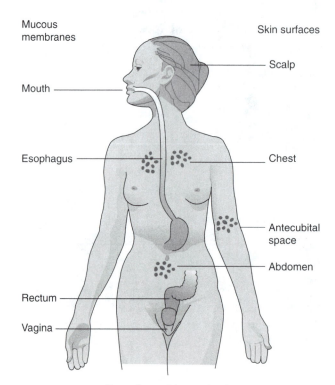

Sites of pemphigus vulgaris.

Report 10: Bess Martin was sent to Radiology for an x-ray of her chest because she had been experiencing pain and shortness of breath.

Words & Phonetic Pronunciations		Definitions
lateral	(lăt´ĕr-ăl)	pertaining to a side
PA		posteroanterior (a direction)
pleuritic chest pain	(ploo-rĭt´ĭk)	chest pain due to inflammation of the pleura

Report 11: Carol White had a baby 6 months ago and has had some urinary tract and vaginal problems in the interim. She comes in today for a general check-up and to discuss these problems with her PCP.

Words & Phonetic Pronunciations

Definitions

abortus [L.]   (ah-bŏr´tŭs)   a fetus weighing less than 500 g (17 oz) or being of less than 20 completed weeks' gestational age at the time of expulsion from the uterus, having no chance of survival

adnexa   (ăd-nĕk´sah)   appendages or adjunct parts (this word is the same whether singular or plural)

axillary lymphadenopathy   (ăk´sĭ-lār´´ē   disease of lymph glands in the armpit
                              lĭm-făd´´ĕ-nŏp´ah-thē)

bruit [Fr.]   (brwe) (bro͞ot)   a sound or murmur heard on auscultation, especially an abnormal one; usually used in the plural, bruits

DTRs   deep tendon reflexes (noted on exam of the extremities)

dysuria   (dĭs-ū´rē-ah)   painful or difficult urination

gravida 2   (grăv´ĭ-dah)   second pregnancy

P&A   percussion and auscultation (feeling and listening to)

para 1   (păr´ah)   a woman who has produced one viable young regardless of whether the child was living at birth

Premarin®   (prĕm´ah-rĭn)   trade name for estrogen replacement drug for menopause

ROM   range of motion (in relation to the extremities)

RRR   regular rate and rhythm (in relation to the heart)

supraclavicular	(soo˝prah-klah-vĭk´ū-lăr)	situated superior to the clavicle (collar bone)
suprapubic	(soo˝prah-pū´bĭk)	situated superior to the pubic arch
visceromegaly	(vĭs˝ĕr-ō-mĕg´ah-lē)	enlargement of the viscera (internal organs)
Voltaren®	(vōl´tă-rĕn)	trade name for diclofenac sodium, a nonsteroidal anti-inflammatory drug

Report 12: Nicolle Brooks, an elderly female with multiple medical problems, was sent to the gastroenterology specialist for a special examination of her upper GI tract due to a stricture of her esophagus.

Words & Phonetic Pronunciations

Definitions

asymptomatic	(ā´´sĭmp-tō-măt´ĭk)	showing or causing no symptoms
bougie dilatations	(boo´zhē dĭl´´ah-tā´shŭns)	a slender, flexible, hollow or solid, cylindrical instrument for introduction into a tubular organ for the purpose of dilating constricted areas
cisapride	(sĭs´ă-prīd)	treatment for gastroesophageal reflux disease, constipation, and dyspepsia
Demerol®	(děm´ěr-ŏl)	trade name for meperidine hydrochloride, a preoperative drug to sedate and to relieve pain
duodenum	(dū´´ō-dē´nŭm) (dū-ŏd´ě-nŭm)	the first or proximal portion of the small intestine
endoscope	(ěn´dō-skōp)	an instrument for the examination of the interior of a hollow viscus, such as the urinary bladder
esophagogastroduodenoscopy	(ě-sŏf´´ah-gō-găs´´trō-dū´´ŏd-ě-nŏs´kō-pē)	endoscopic examination of the esophagus, stomach, and duodenum
gastroesophageal	(găs´´trō-ě-sŏf´´ah-jē´ăl)	pertaining to the stomach and esophagus
GE		gastroesophageal
LES		lower esophageal sphincter
nasogastric	(nā´´zō-găs´trĭk)	pertaining to the nose and stomach
oropharynx	(ō´´rō-făr´ĭngks)	division of the pharynx that lies between the soft palate and the upper edge of the epiglottis
patent	(pā´těnt)	open, unobstructed, or not closed

patulous	(păt´ū-lŭs)	spreading widely apart; open; distended
pylorus	(pī-lŏr´ŭs)	the distal aperture of the stomach
Versed®	(vĕr-sĕd´)	trade name for midazolam hydrochloride, a drug used for preoperative sedation, before a diagnostic or radiographic procedure

Report 13: Lynda Shoemaker was sent to Cardiology for an echocardiogram because of chest pain and shortness of breath.

Words & Phonetic Pronunciations		Definitions
2-D data		two-dimensional information found on echocardiography
aortic stenosis	(ā-ŏr´tĭk stĕ-nō´sĭs)	narrowing of the orifice of the aortic valve
Doppler	(dŏp´lĕr)	brand name of the instrument (used in radiology)
color flow imaging		images in color rather than black and white, a radiology term
excursion	(ĕk-skŭr´zhŭn)	movements occurring from a normal, or rest, position of a movable part in performance of a function
interventricular	(ĭn´´tĕr-vĕn-trĭk´ū-lăr)	situated between ventricles
M-mode data		information obtained on a diagnostic ultrasound procedure (radiology)
sclerotic	(sklĕ-rŏt´ĭk)	hard or hardening
septal	(sĕp´tăl)	pertaining to a septum (a dividing wall or partition)
ventricular	(vĕn-trĭk´ū-lăr)	pertaining to a ventricle (one of the lower chambers of the heart)

Report 14: John J. Wagner, a heart patient, had a recent hospital admission. He comes to his PCP for a regular check-up and to discuss the possibility of a transplant.

Words & Phonetic Pronunciations		Definitions
afebrile	(ā-fĕb´rĭl)	without fever
bibasilar crackles	(bī-băs´ĭ-lăr)	abnormal sounds (crackles) heard primarily during inhalation in the bases of both lungs
bilaterally	(bī-lăt´ĕr-ăl-ē)	pertaining to both sides
Capoten®	(kăp´ō-tĕn)	trade name for captopril, an ACE inhibitor drug used for hypertension
Cardene®	(kahr´dēn)	trade name for nicardipine hydrochloride, a calcium channel blocker drug used for angina and hypertension
cardiomyopathy	(kăr´´dē-ō-mī-ŏp´ah-thē)	a general diagnostic term designating primary noninflammatory disease of the heart muscle
CHF		congestive heart failure
Coumadin®	(koo´mah-dĭn)	trade name for warfarin sodium, an anticoagulant drug
Ecotrin®	(ĕk´ō-trĭn)	trade name for acetylsalicylic acid, a nonsteroidal anti-inflammatory drug
ischemic	(ĭs-kē´mĭk)	pertaining to, or affected with, ischemia (deficiency of blood in a part)
Lasix®	(lā´sĭks)	trade name for furosemide, a diuretic drug
Nitro-Dur®	(nī´tră-dŭr)	trade name for nitroglycerin, an antianginal drug
prothrombin	(prō-thrŏm´bĭn)	a factor in the blood plasma that combines with calcium to form thrombin during blood clotting

tachycardia   (tăk´´ē-kăr´dē-ah)   excessive rapidity in the action of the
                                                           heart

VQ scan   ventilation-perfusion scan (for
                                                           demonstrating defects in the lungs)

Report 15: Barbara Ann Richards is a young woman who was referred to Psychiatry because of a bad experience with drug abuse and some suicidal tendencies.

Words & Phonetic Pronunciations   ## Definitions

chemotherapy   (kē´´mō-thĕr´ah-pē)   treatment of disease by chemical agents

EMS   Emergency Medical Service

GAF Scale   Global Assessment of Functional Scale, a psychiatric term

psychotherapy   (sī´´kō-thĕr´ah-pē)   treatment of mental disorders and behavioral disturbances

Report 16: Jim Wilson was referred to Dermatology because of a recurrent and persistent rash.

Words & Phonetic Pronunciations

Definitions

Words & Phonetic Pronunciations		Definitions
autosomal	(aw´tō-sōm-ăl)	any ordinary paired chromosome alike in males and females, as distinguished from sex chromosomes
Darier's disease	(dăr´ē-āz)	urtication and itching occurring on rubbing the lesions of urticaria pigmentosa
genodermatosis	(jē´´nō-děr´´mah-tō´sĭs)	a genetically determined disorder of the skin, usually generalized
keratosis follicularis	(kěr´´ah-tō´sĭs fō-lĭk-ū-lăr´ĭs)	a slowly progressive autosomal dominant disorder of keratinization characterized by pinkish to tan or skin-colored papules on the seborrheic areas of the body that coalesce to form plaques, which may become crusted and secondarily infected
keratosis pilaris	(kěr´´ah-tō´sĭs pē-lăr´ĭs)	a condition in which hyperkeratosis is limited to the hair follicles

Report 17: Joseph Patrick, an elderly male with multiple medical problems, was referred to Urology because of his retention of blood clots after manipulation of his Foley catheter.

Words & Phonetic Pronunciations

Definitions

adenocarcinoma	(ăd˝ĕ-nō-kăr˝sĭ-nō´mah)	carcinoma derived from glandular tissue
ASHD		arteriosclerotic heart disease
bilateral orchiectomy	(bī-lăt´ĕr-ăl ŏr˝kē-ĕk´tō-mē)	pertaining to the excision of both testes
BUN		blood urea nitrogen (a lab test)
metastatic disease	(mĕt˝ah-stăt´ĭk)	the transfer of disease from one organ or part to another not directly connected with it
PSA		prostate-specific antigen (a lab test to identify cancer of the prostate)
Septra®	(sĕp´tră)	trade name for trimethoprim and sulfamethoxazole, an antibiotic drug
transurethral resection	(trăns˝ū-rē´thrăl rē-sĕk´shŭn)	excision of a portion or all of an organ performed through the urethra, usually the prostate
Urecholine®	(ū˝rē-kō´lĭn)	trade name for bethanechol chloride, or urinary antispasmodic drug

Report 18: George Nandor has had difficulty sleeping and was referred for a sleep study. Patients
are kept overnight for these studies, sometimes for two nights, as Mr. Nandor was.

Words & Phonetic Pronunciations   Definitions

Word	Pronunciation	Definition
apnea	(ăp´nē-ah)	cessation of breathing
electrocardiogram	(ē-lĕk˝trō-kăr´dē-ō-grăm)	a graphic tracing of the variations in electrical potential caused by the excitation of the heart muscle and detected at the body surface, abbreviated ECG or EKG
electro-oculographic	(ē-lĕk˝trō-ŏk˝ū-lō-grăf´ĭk)	pertaining to the electroencephalographic (brain wave) tracings made by moving the eyes a constant distance between two fixation points
electroencephalographic	(ē-lĕk˝trō-ĕn-sĕf´ah-lo-grăf-ĭk)	pertaining to the recording of the electric currents developed by the brain, abbreviated EEG
electromyogram	(ē-lĕk˝trō-mī´ō-grăm)	the record obtained by recording the extracellular activity of skeletal muscles at rest, during voluntary contractions, and during electrical stimulation, abbreviated EMG
hypopnea	(hī-pŏp´nē-ah)	abnormal decrease in the depth and rate of the respiratory movements
hypoxemia	(hī˝pŏk-sē´mē-ah)	deficient oxygenation of the blood
myoclonic	(mī˝ō-klō´nĭk)	pertaining to shocklike contractions of a portion of a muscle, an entire muscle, or a group of muscles
oximetry	(ŏk-sĭm´ē-trē)	determination of the oxygen saturation of arterial blood using an oximeter
pharyngeal	(făr-rĭn´jē-ăl)	pertaining to the pharynx (throat)

polysomnography   (pŏl´´ē-sŏm-nŏg´rah-fē)   the polygraphic recording during sleep of multiple physiologic variables both directly and indirectly related to the state and stages of sleep, to assess possible biologic causes of sleep disorders

somnolence   (sŏm´nō-lĕns)   sleepiness; also unnatural drowsiness

thermistor   (thĕr-mĭs´tŏr)   a thermometer whose impedance varies with the ambient temperature and so is able to measure extremely small changes in temperature

uvula   (ū´vū-lah)   a pendent, fleshy mass extended from the soft palate

Report 19: Leslie Arispe is an elderly female who has dementia and depression and is suicidal. She was referred to Psychiatry for examination and for treatment recommendations.

Words & Phonetic Pronunciations

Definitions

adenopathy	(ăd´´ĕ-nŏp´ah-thē)	enlargement of the glands
arcus senilis	(ăr´kŭs sĕn-ĭl´ŭs)	curved or bow-like corneae
Ativan®	(ăt´ĭ-văn)	trade name for lorazepam, an antianxiety drug
benzodiazepines	(bĕn´´zō-dī-ăz´ĕ-pēns)	class of drugs used to treat anxiety and insomnia
bilateral	(bī-lăt´ĕr-ăl)	pertaining to both sides
bradycardia	(brăd´´ē-kăr´dē-ah)	slowness of the heartbeat
cholecystectomy	(kō´´lē-sĭs-tĕk´tō-mē)	surgical removal of the gallbladder
cyanosis	(sī´´ah-nō´sĭs)	a bluish discoloration of the skin due to excessive concentration of reduced hemoglobin in the blood
dementia	(dē-mĕn´shē-ah)	an organic mental syndrome characterized by a general loss of intellectual abilities involving impairment of memory, judgment, and abstract thinking as well as changes in personality
Depakote®	(dĕp´ă-kōt)	trade name for divalproex sodium, a drug used to treat seizures
dysuria	(dĭs-ūr´rē-ah)	painful or difficult urination
EKG, ECG		electrocardiogram
flurazepam	(floor-ăz´ĕ-păm)	nonbarbiturate drug used for insomnia
gait	(gāt)	manner or style of walking

Haldol®	(hăl´dŏl)	trade name for haloperidol, an antipsychotic drug
hepatosplenomegaly	(hĕp´´ah-tō-splē´´nō-mĕg´ah-lē)	enlargement of the liver and spleen
hypercholesterolemia	(hī´´pĕr-kō-lĕs´´tĕr-ŏl-ē´mē-ah)	excess of cholesterol in the blood
hyperglycemia	(hī´´pĕr-glī-sē´mē-ah)	abnormally increased content of glucose (sugar) in the blood
hypotensive	(hī´´pō-tĕn´sĭv)	abnormally low blood pressure
hypovolemia	(hī´pō-vō-le´mē-ah)	abnormally decreased volume of circulating fluid (plasma) in the body
hysterectomy	(hĭs´´tĕ-rĕck´tō-mē)	the operation of excising the entire uterus, performed either through the abdominal wall or through the vagina
ketoacidosis	(kē´´tō-ăs´´ĭ-dō´sĭs)	acidosis accompanied by the accumulation of ketone bodies in the body tissues and fluids
lithium	(lĭth´ē-ŭm)	drug used for manic-depressive disorders
Paxil®	(păx´ŭl)	trade name for paroxetine hydrochloride, an antidepressant drug
Premarin®	(prēm´ah-rĭn)	trade name for estrogen replacement drug for menopause
salpingo-oophorectomy	(săl-pĭng´´gō-ō´´ŏf-ō-rĕk´tō-mē)	surgical removal of a uterine tube and ovary
somnolent	(sŏm´nō-lĕnt)	affected with somnolence; sleepy
trazodone	(trā´zō-dōn)	antidepressant drug
urinalysis	(ū´´rĭ-năl´ĭ-sĭs)	physical, chemical, or microscopic analysis or examination of urine

Vasotec®	(văs´ō-těk)	trade name for enalapril maleate, an inhibitor drug used for hypertension
verapamil	(věr´´ah-păm´ĭl)	drug used for angina, arrythmias, and hypertension; also used for migraine headaches
vulvectomy	(vŭl-věk´tō-mē)	excision of the vulva

Report 20: B. Christine Anello is a young woman in the second trimester of a difficult pregnancy with massive fetal deformities. She is seen by both an Obstetrics specialist and a Geneticist. See Illustrations on page 186.

Words & Phonetic Pronunciations

		Definitions
acetylcholinesterase	(ăs´´ĕ-tĭl-ko´´lĭn-ĕs´tĕr-ās)	an enzyme; it is found in the central nervous system
amniocentesis	(ăm´´nē-ō-sĕn-tē´sĭs)	percutaneous transabdominal puncture of the uterus to obtain amniotic fluid
Bartholin's gland	(băr´tō-lĭnz)	one of the two small bodies on either side of the vaginal orifice
bilirubin	(bĭl´´ĭ-roo´bĭn)	a bile pigment
chlamydia	(klah-mĭd´ē-ah)	a common sexually transmitted disease caused by the *Chlamydia* bacteria
Cleocin®	(klē´ō-sĭn)	trade name for clindamycin, an antibiotic
epithelialized	(ĕp´´ĭ-thē´lē-ăl-īzd)	healed by the growth of epithelium (skin) over a denuded surface
gamma GT	(găm´ah)	gamma-glutamyl transferase; sometimes GGT (a lab test)
Gardnerella	(gărd´´nĕr-ĕl´ah)	bacteria found in the normal female genital tract and also as a major cause of bacterial vaginitis
hepatitis	(hĕp´´ah-tī´tĭs)	inflammation of the liver
hydrocephalus	(hī´´drō-sĕf´ah-lŭs)	an accumulation of cerebrospinal fluid within the skull
Imuran®	(ĭm´ū-răn)	trade name for azathioprine, an immunosuppressant; used to prevent transplant rejection
jaundice	(jawn´dĭs)	a syndrome characterized by hyperbilirubinemia and deposition of bile pigment in the skin, mucous membranes and sclerae with resulting yellow appearance of the patient's skin and eyes

LMP   last menstrual period

myocardial infarction   (mī´´ō-kăr´dē-ăl   gross necrosis of the myocardium as a
                               ĭn-fărk´shŭn)   result of interruption of the blood supply
                                                         to the area (heart attack)

neonatal   (nē´´ō-ña´tăl)   pertaining to a newborn infant

primigravida   (prī´´mĭ-grăv´ĭ-dah)   a woman pregnant for the first time

RPR   rapid plasma reagin (a lab test for
                                                         syphilis)

SGOT   serum glutamic oxaloacetic transaminase
                                                         (a lab test)

SGPT   serum glutamic-pyruvic transaminase (a
                                                         lab test)

Skene's glands   (skēnz)   glands of the female urethra

thoracolumbar   (thō´´rah-kō-lŭm´băr)   pertaining to the thoracic and lumbar
                                                         parts of the spine

U/L   units per liter (a measurement)

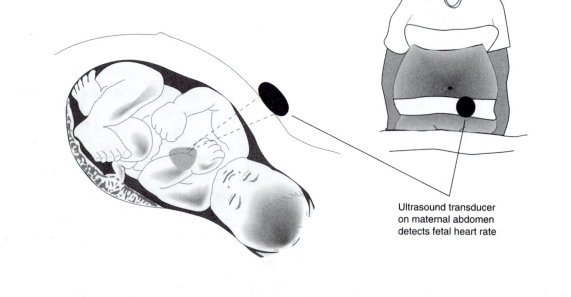

Ultrasound transducer
on maternal abdomen
detects fetal heart rate

Skill-Building Exercises

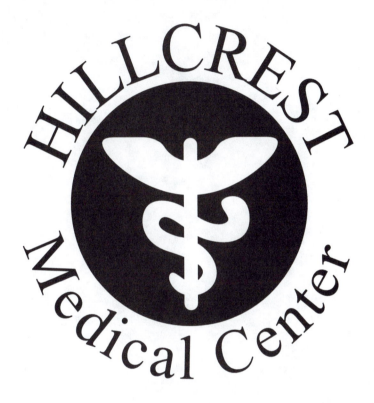

CROSSWORD PUZZLE 1

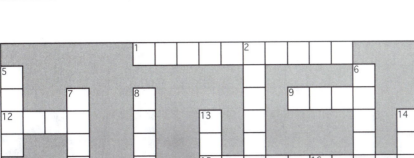

ACROSS

1. within the skull
3. prefix for behind, backward
9. prefix for many
10. not breathing
12. prefix for near, beside
15. inflammation of many nerves
17. prefix for bad, painful, difficult
19. prefix for small
21. pertaining to two joints
22. through the skin
24. without oxygen
26. a newborn infant
28. prefix for above, upon
30. prefix for one half, partly
31. near the esophagus
32. uniting together
33. between the ribs

DOWN

2. inflammation of one half of the tongue
4. good digestion
5. prefix for deficient, below
6. prefix for above, excessive
7. total hysterectomy
8. slow heartbeat
11. affecting both sides
13. double vision
14. prefix for before
16. removal
18. painful menstrual flow
20. situated above a kidney
23. prefix for within
25. before the onset of fever
27. out of normal position
29. complete separation

Student _____

ACROSS

1. suture of the intestine
8. a discharge from the ear
12. absence of oxygen
14. combining form for cheek
15. formation of bone marrow
18. pertaining to the mouth
19. combining form for joint
21. combining form for stone, calculus
25. abnormal dryness
26. combining form for sacrum
28. pain in the coccyx
29. any disease of the skull

DOWN

2. hemorrhage from a kidney
3. pertaining to the kidney
4. surgical repair of an artery
5. combining form for arm
6. combining form for side
7. pertaining to the lips and tongue
9. combining form for tooth
10. constriction of the stomach
11. blood in the urine
13. combining form for nerve
16. combining form for pulse
17. combining form for mouth
20. incision of a joint
22. destruction of tissue
23. any disease of the bursa
24. combining form for internal organs
27. an x-ray of the urinary bladder

CROSSWORD PUZZLE 3

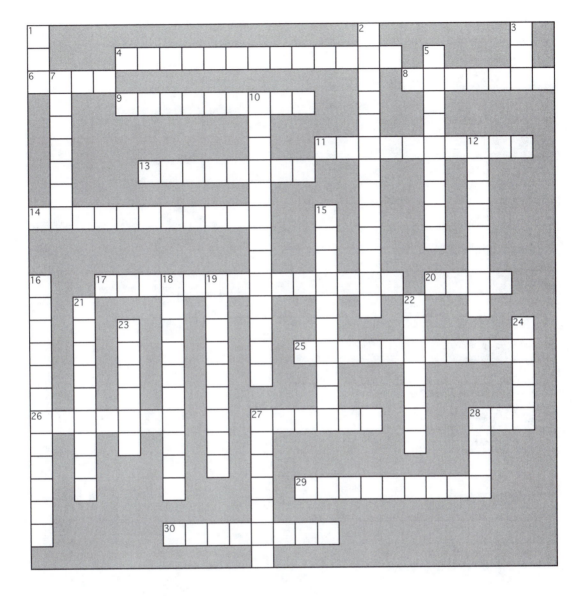

ACROSS

4. suture of a hernia
6. suffix for an instrument used to cut bone
8. difficult breathing
9. surgical creation of a new opening in the colon
11. enlargement of extremities
13. inflammation of a bone
14. pain in the stomach
17. drooping of the eyelid
20. suffix for inflammation
25. excessive vomiting
26. absence of the sense of smell
27. suffix for irrigation, washing
28. suffix for tumor
29. discharge of the menses
30. pertaining to the chest

DOWN

1. suffix for specialist
2. the formation of cartilage
3. suffix for little, small
5. bad digestion
7. pain in the ear

10. study of the eye
12. lack of strength
15. spitting blood
16. softening of bone
18. excessive eating
19. a minute arterial branch
21. dimming of vision
22. suffix for treatment
23. suffix for new opening
24. suffix for smell
27. pertaining to the heart
28. suffix for vision

CROSSWORD PUZZLE 4

Student _____

ACROSS

3. overgrowth of an organ
4. performed through a vein
8. surgical removal of a polyp
10. enlargement of the heart
12. occurring after a surgical procedure
14. yielding something abundantly
15. throat
18. without fever
22. pertaining to the cheek
23. enlargement of the viscera
24. analysis of urine

DOWN

1. pertaining to the femur
2. persisting over a long period of time
4. fast and slow heartbeat
5. a brief loss of consciousness
6. within the trachea
7. inflammation of the liver
9. the rough white outer coat of the eyeball
11. enlargement of the thyroid gland
13. located beneath the tongue
16. pertaining to the uterus and sacrum
17. difficult breathing
19. a bluish discoloration
20. difficult breathing except in an upright position
21. falling down of a part or an organ

Student _____

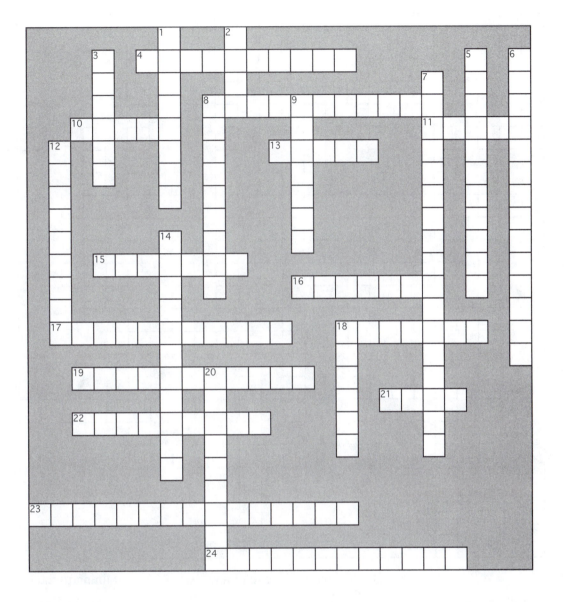

ACROSS

4. inflammation of the oral mucosa
8. study of the skin
10. pertaining to the kidney
11. lying face downward
13. a sound or murmur heard on auscultation
15. painful urination
16. widely distributed
17. any joint disease
18. relating to the principal artery of the neck
19. within a vein
21. to cast out as waste matter
22. inflammation of the joints
23. surgical removal of the gallbladder
24. enlargement of the spleen

DOWN

1. the cause(s) or origin of a disease
2. an abnormal respiratory sound heard on auscultation
3. to remove part of an organ or tissue
5. abnormally low blood pressure
6. situated between two contiguous vertebrae
7. abnormally increased coloration
8. difficulty in swallowing
9. wasting away
12. blood in the urine
14. pertaining to the lumbar vertebrae and sacrum
18. having a rounded, somewhat elevated surface
20. inflammation of the intestine

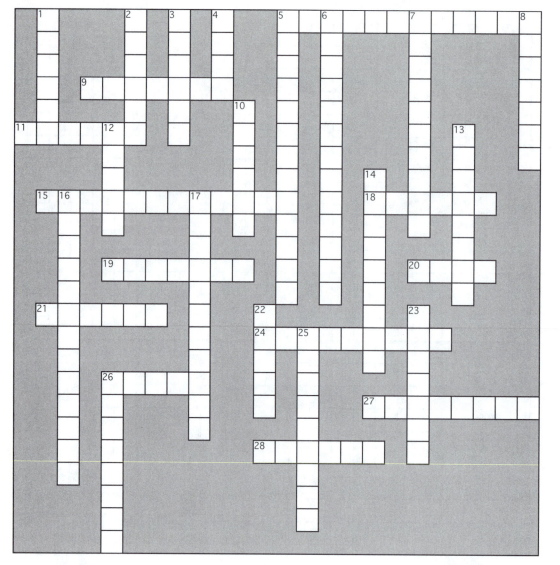

ACROSS

5. inflammation of the brain
9. of the nature or quality of bone
11. pertaining to the middle
15. pertaining to the ribs and diaphragm
18. armpit
19. pertaining to the heart
20. manner or style of walking
21. vomiting
24. a minute arterial branch
26. a finger or toe
27. the study of cells
28. the bottom or base of anything

DOWN

1. irrigation of an organ
2. pertaining to the back
3. pertaining to the veins
4. medical jargon; shortened version of segmented neutrophils
5. pertaining to within the bronchi
6. inflammation of the gallbladder
7. variation from the normal rhythm of the heartbeat
8. pertaining to the sternum
10. black vomit
12. having a short, severe course
13. the perception of two images of a single object
14. inflammation of the stomach
16. inflammation of bone caused by a pyogenic organism
17. disease of the retina
22. heat
23. pertaining to the sole of the foot
25. pertaining to a tendon
26. the first portion of the small intestine

Proofreading Exercise 1

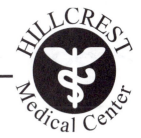

Student _____ (25 errors)

DEATG SUMMARY

Patient Name: Teiko Sun

Hospital No.: 46901

Admitted: 08/17/- - - -

Deceased: 08/20/- - - - at 4:30 p.m.

Consultations: None.

Procedures: Proctoscopy.

This 75-year-old Asian femail patient was admitted through the ER with a cute massive rectal blooding of unknown origin, possibly diverticulitis; congestive heart failure in mild exacerbation; chromic renal failure, worsening since the day before admission, with dehidrition; and cronic atrial fribillation.

Emergency proctoscopy was done in the GI suite immediately after leaving the ER, which reveal only clodded blood without a source for the bleeding. Colonoskopie was scheduled but then later canceled do to pour bowel preparation and extreem weakness on the part of the patient.

A nuclear-tagged red blunt cell bleeding study was performed in order to localise the bleeding cite in case of the necessity of emergency bowel surgery, but this proved to show no specific source of the bleeding. The bleeding apparently stopped spontaneously. Homoglobin and hemocrat descended to a nadir of 11.9 and 33.7 respectfully the day after admission.

The patient's chronic renal flailure worsened steadily with increasing creatinine and BON and decreasing CO_2. At the request of the family no hemodialysis was dun. Her chronic renal failure worsened further and eventually he died at 4:30 p.m., three days after admission.

_____
Sangita Mehtapur, M.D.

SM:xx
D:08/20/- - - -
T:08/23/- - - -

Proofreading Exercise 2

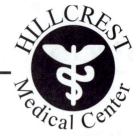

Student _____ **(26 errors)**

HISTORY AND PHYSICAL EXAMINATION

Patient Name: Patrick Platt

Hospital No.: 77103

Room No.: 560

Date of Admission: 08/30/- - - -

Admitting Physician: William Payne, M.D.

Admitting Diagnosis: Rule out fracture of left arm.

CHIEF COMPLAINT: Pain and swelling, left upper arm.

HISTORY OF PRESENT ILLNESS: The patient is an elderly female who fell four days prior to admission. He noted immediate pain and swelling in the area just below his left elbow. He presented to the emergency roomf or treatment.

PAST HISTORY: Past illness includes Whooping cough as a child. Tonsillectomy in 1947. No known allergies to medications.

FAMILY HISTORY: No hereditary disorders noted. Mother and father are deceased. Two brothers are alive and well. One sister has adult set diabetes mellitus.

SOCIAL HISTORY: The married and has two children. His wife does not work outside the home.

PHYSICAL EXAMINATION: GENERAL: The patient is a well-developed, well nourished male who appears to be in moderate distress with pain and swelling in the upper left arm. Vital sign: Blood pressure 140/90, temperature 98.3, pulse 97, respiration 18.

HEENT: Head normal, no lesions. Eyes: Arcus senilis,both eyes. Ears: Impacted cerumen, left ear. Nose: Clear. Mouth: Dentures fit well, no lesions.

NECK: Normal range of motion in all directs.

(Continued)

HISTORY AND PHYSICAL EXAMINATION
Patient Name: Patrick Platt
Hospital No.: 77103
Page 2

INTEGUMENTARY: Psoriatic lesion, right thigh, approximately 1 mL in diameter.

CHEST: Clear breath sounds bilaterally. No rales or rhonchi noted.

HEART: Normal sinus rhythm. There is a holosystolic murmur. No friction rubs noted.

ABDOMEN: Normal bowl sounds. Liver, kidneys, and spleen are normal to palpitation.

GENITALIA: Tests normally descended bilaterally.

RECTAL: Prostrate 2+ and benign.

EXTREMITIES: Pain and swelling noted above the left elbow, other upper extremities normal. No cyanosis or clubbing. The legs demonstrate 2+ pitting edema to the knees.

NEUROLOGIC: Cranial nerves II-XII intact, Memory intact, Sensation intact to light tough.

ASSESSMENT AND PLAN: The patinet was sent for plain film of the left arm, which revealed a fractured of the left humorous. The fracture was reduce in the emergency room. X-ray revealed anatomic alignment.

He was released to home with a perscription for a nonsteroidal anti-inflammatory and instructions to elevate his arm. He will be follow in the office in three days.

PROGNOSIS: Good.

_____

William Payne, M.D.

WM:xx
D:08/30/- - - -
T:09/01/- - - -

Proofreading Exercise 3

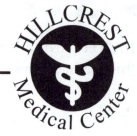

HILLCREST Medical Center

Student _____ **(24 errors)**

REQUEST FOR CONSULTATION

Patient Name: David Moore

Hospital No.: 24601

Consultant: Carl M. Martin, M.D., Gastroenterology

Requesting Physician: Donald Burns, M.D., Family Medicine

Date: 03/15/- - - -

Reason for Consultation: Please evaluate GI distress.

I was ask to see this 23-year-old male in consultation because of unremitting nausea, diarrhoea, vomitting, abdominal pain, dizziness, and low-grade fever. The patient has a poor appetite but report no weight loss. He has noted some postprandial cramping, midepigastric pain, and unremitting diarrhea but no blood in the stols. He states he is "better" but he still has some dizziness.

Initial treatment consisted of I.V. fluids and control of electrolites. Thereafter, the patient was progressedto clear fluids and soft diet. He has done well on this regiment; however, his dizziness has persisted. Fever has resolve.

On admission, the patients' lab data revealed CBC with hematocrit of 42, hemoglobin 25 with differential of neutrophils 52%, bands 9%, lymphocytes 25%, monocytes 5%, basophils none. Serum electrolytes were normal. Potassium was low at 3.3, BUN/creatinine ratio was normal. Glucase was within normal range. Stool studies was normal. Urine analysis within normal limit except for 8-10 WBCs. Specific gravy was 1.025.

On exam I find the patient to be lethargic and uncomfortable with mild nausea and dizziness. He prefers to keep his eyes closed. On examination of the throat, I find no nystagmus. There is pallor to the skin, and he seems cool to the touch. Upon standing by the bedside, the patient is unsteady. Although he resists to walking, when he attempts to walk, his gate is halting, and he tends to fall to the left side. Abdomen is flat and nontender. Bowel sounds are WNL. Rectal deferred.

(Continued)

REQUEST FOR CONSULTATION
Patient Name: David Moore
Hospital No.:   24601
Page 2

RECOMMENDATIONS: I think we should continue low-key treat of this elderly gentlemen. Because of the symptoms of dizziness on admission, we may want to consider a CT scan to rule out a intracerebral bleed or subdural hematoma. My opinion at this time is that we are dealing with a resolving about of gastritis.

Thank you for asking me to see this patient. I will be glad to follow him with you throughout his hospitle stay.

_____

Carl M. Martin, M.D.

CMM:xx
D:03/15/- - - -
T:03/16/- - - -

Proofreading Exercise 4

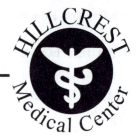

Student _____ (21 errors)

DISCHARGE SUMMARY

Patinet Name: Jack Richardson

Hospital No.: 15790

Admitted: 07/04/- - - -

Discharged: 07/16/- - - -

Consultations: None.

Procedures: Open reduction, internal fixation of fractures.

Complications: None.

Admitting Diagnosis: Multiple trauma from motor vehicle accident, brought in through emergency room.

HISTORY: The patient is a 31-year-old caucasian male which was involved in a MVA approximate two hours prior to admission. On admission he was noted to have an unstable pelvis and a traumatic laceration through the left perineum, indicative of an open fracture. The patient also had a left femoral head dislocation. X-rays of the left foot and ankle revealed a severely comminuted fracture, left angle. Patient was admitted ot general surgery service to rule out intra-abdominal injury.

HOSPITAL COARSE: The day following admittion patient underwent open reduction, internal fixation of his fractured pelvis and ankle fractured. He did well following surgery and was ambulating on postoperative day two. He began rehabilitation in the physical therapy department and will continue physiotherapy followed discharge. He remain afebrile throught his hospital stay. On discharge all wounds were healing without complication and were clean and dry. There were no sighs of infection. A short-leg caste was applied to the left leg prior to discharge.

DISCHARGE MEDICATIONS: Tylenol No, 3 one p.o. q. 4 to 6 h.

DISCHARGE INSTRUCTIONS: Patient is to be seen in the orthopaedic clinic in one week for would check and x-rays of the pelvis and left ankle. He will be seen in general surgery service in two weeks. Activities as tolerant, elevate the leg, call if he has a problem prior to his follow-up visit.

(Continued)

DISCHARGE SUMMARY
Patinet Name: Jack Richardson
Hospital No.: 15790
Page 2

DISCHARGE DIAGNOSES: 1. Comminuded fracture, left ankle.
                              2. Fractured pelvis.

_____

Ping Wu, M.D.

PW:xx
D:08/02/- - - -
T:08/03/- - - -

Proofreading Exercise 5

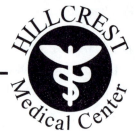

Student _____ (16 errors)

DISCHARGE SUMMARY

Patient Name: Hank Babcock

Hospital No.: 65227

Admitted: 01/14/- - - -

Discharged: 01/18/- - - -

Consultationz: Dr. Jose Medina, M.D., Surgeon

Procedures: Appendectomy.

Complications: Nine.

Admitting Diagnosis: Rule out acute appendicitis.

This is a 45-year-old black man seen in my office on January 14 with the onset of acute abdominal pain at 10 am that day. He was admitted directly to hte hospital with a diagnosis of probable acute appendicitis.

LABORATORY DATA: Serm amylase was normal at 64. Cultures of peritoneal fluid at the time of discharged showed no growth. CBC performed as a follow-up on January 16 showed a white account of 12,400 (decreased from 21,000 on January 14). Hemoglobin to day is 12 (decreased from 15.5 on January 14). Preop laboratory data was performed in the office prior to admission. The reminder of the values were within the reference range for our facility.

HOSPITAL COURSE: The patient was admitted and surgical consultatin was obtained from Dr. Medina. The patient was taken to surgery the evening of admission where acute appendicitis with a small perforation was find. Pathology confirmed acute appendicitis. The patient convalecsed without difficulties, although he did have a low-grade fever of 99.9F until January 17.

He was discharged on the following medication: Darvocet-N 100 one q. 6 h. p.r.n. pain and Keflex 500 mg p.o. q. 6 h. for three days. Diet and activities at the time of discharge is as tolerated.

DISCHARGE DIAGNOSIS: Acute suppurative appendicitis.

(Continued)

DISCHARGE SUMMARY
Patient Name: Hank Babcock
Hospital No.: 65227
Page 2

DISPOSITION: He will be seen by Dr. Medina in five days. He will be seen in my office in six weeks to be evaluated four possible hypercholesterolemia and possible hypothyroidism.

_____

Ruth Ellis, M.D.

RE:xx
D:01/20/- - - -
T:01/22/- - - -

Proofreading Exercise 6

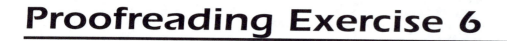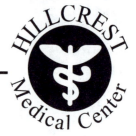

Student _____ (15 errors)

RADIOLOGY REPORT

Patient Name: Wayne Masten

Hospital No.: 70991

X-ray No.: 94-81938

Admitting Physician: Hannah Sommers, M.D.

Procedure: PA and lateral chest.

Date: 12/21/- - - -

CLINICAL INFORMATION: Weakness, lethargy. Rule out AIDS, *Pneumocystis* pneumonia. Patient has difficulty breathin and has been unable to gain wait. No IV drug abuse but she admits to promisecuity. Old films are unavailable for comparison.

Findings of underling COPD are noted. The heart size appears normal. The pulmonary vessels, where they can be evaluated, appear unremarkable. Their is no evidence of plural effusion.

Extensive interstitial infiltrates are presnet throughout both lungs. The findings are most consistant with diffused bilateral interstitial pneumonia. I presume we are dealing predominantly with interstitial fibrosis. The lung sare hyperinflated, and there are emphysematous changes in both upper lobe, more prominent on the right.

IMPRESSION: 1. COPD with bullous emphysema.
                2. Sever diffuse interstitial lung disease, most likely interstitial fibrosis.
                3. *Pneumocystis carinii* pneumonia should be considered in the differential diagnosis.

_____

Anne J. Tulsa, M.D.

ATJ:xx
D:12/21/- - - -
T:12/21/- - - -

204

Proofreading Exercise 7

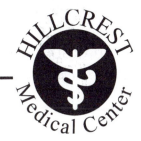

Student _____ (18 errors)

REQUEST FOR CONSULTATION

Patient Name: Victor Peterson

Hospital No.: 97357

Consultant: Mary Wells, M.D., Gastroenterology Services

Requesting Physician: Erik Lunderman, M.D., Pulmonary/Respiratory Services

Date: 10/16/- - - -

Reason for Consultation: Please evaluate RUQ abdominal pain.

HISTORY: This patient, a 58-year-old male, been seen at the request of his pulmonary/respiratory physician on Friday, October 16, has been admitted to the hospital for elective thorocotomy and decortication for suspected mesothelioma. The patient has a long history of asbestos expo sure, having difficulty with shoulder and arm pain, with the diagnosis of mesothelioma. Two days ago he developed right upper quadrant abdominal pain. The patient has never experienced this type of dyscomfort; he has had no history of acid peptic disease, no known cholelithiasis. He denies fever, chills, hemituria, disurea, or frequency.

PHYSICAL EXAMINATION being done at this time is limited to the abdomin where bowel sounds are present and normal. There are no discreet mass felt. There is fullness in the right upper quadrant, and the patient does exhibit some minimal tenderness to palpation in the right upper quadrant. The patient has being a febrile. Ultrasound of the gall bladder does show cholelithiasis with a borderling common duct.

DISCUSSION: At the present time the patient is known to have stones. I suspect his discomfort is from either an episodes of cholecystitis nor choledocholithiasis. I would suspect that livor function studies may be helpful in suggesting the presents of choledocholithiasis. We will make arrangements for the LFTs and possible sphincterotomy.

IMPRESSION: 1. Status post resection of mesothelioma.
                2. Cholelithiasis, rule out choledocholithiasis.

(Continued)

DISCHARGE SUMMARY
Patient Name: Victor Peterson
Hospital No.: 97357
Page 2

Thank you very much for allowing us to participate in the care of your patient. We will follow along with you as necessary.

_____

Mary Wells, M.D.

MW:xx
D:10/16/- - - -
T:10/17/- - - -

Proofreading Exercise 8

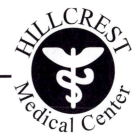

Student _____ **(21 errors)**

HISTORY AND PHYSICAL EXAMINATION

Patient Name: Maria Elena Ramirez

Hospital No.: 15837

Room No.: 532

Date of Admission: 10/20/- - - -

Admitting Physician: Hal Seggerman, M.D.

Admitting Diagnosis: Rule out adenomyosis of uterus.

CHIEF COMPLAIN: Exceedingly heavy and painfully menses.

PRESENT ILLNESS: Patient is a 35-year-old, mildly obese Hispanic female, gravida 5, para 4-1-0-4, whose younger child is 13 years old. Patient states that over the past one years or so she has had increasing difficulty with moodiness, depression, generalized fatigue, weight gain, and bloating premenstrually. The symptoms described preceed her menses by about a weak. She was seen by another physician and diagnosed as having menstrual endometrium.

PAST SURGICAL HISTORY: She has had DNCs on two occasions five or six years ago for what sounds like menorrhagia/metrorrhagia. A sterilization procedure was done afterbirth of her last child.

ALLERGIES/PAST HISTORY/MEDICATIONS: The patient is allergic to <u>Ergotrate</u> an <u>iodine</u>, especially in the forum of IVP die. Her only medication at present is Motrin, used p.r.n. menstrual cramps. She has had the usual childhood diseases with no sequelae, no serious adult illnesses, no similar problems in her remote passed.

PHYSICAL EXAMINATION: VITAL SIGN: Completely within normal limits. HEENT: Normocephalic. PERRLA. NECK: No crepitus. Trachea is midline. No JVD. BREASTS are pendulous with a monilial appearing rash between the breasts. No masses, tenderness, or discharge. Areola are darkly pigmented. ABDOMEN: Fatty abdominal apron with a well-heeled scar at the sight of her sterilization procedure. No hepatosplenomegaly. Positive bowel sounds. PELVIC/RECTAL: Introduction of speculum reveals the cervix to be multiparous and clean. No vaginal wall lesions are noted. On by manual exam, uterus is exquisitely tender to compression and is retroversion in position.

(Continued)

HISTORY AND PHYSICAL EXAMINATION
Patient Name: Maria Elena Ramirez
Hospital No.: 15837
Page 2

Adnexa are negative for masses but are moderately tender. BUS negative. Rectal exam confirmatory with some internal and external hemorrhoid. SKIN: Patient has had some itching between her breasts and on her inner thighs due to apparent Monilia. NEUROLOGIC: No focale deficits.

IMPRESSING: 1. Cyclic edema inadequately compensated.
                2. Probable adenomyosis of the uterus.
                3. Monilia.
                4. Internal and external hemorrhoids.

_____

Hal Seggerman, M.D.

HS:xx
D:10/20/- - - -
T:10/21/- - - -

Proofreading Exercise 9

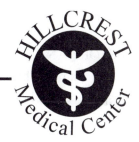

Student _____ (17 errors)

HISTORY AND PHYSICAL EXAMINATION

Patient Name: Christina Youngblood

Hospital No.: 71210

Room No.: 418

Date of Admission: 06/24/- - - -

Admitting Physician: Cynthia Richards, M.D.

Admitting Diagnosis: Cystocele, prolapsed uterus, B9 cyst of vulva.

CHIEF COMPLAINT: Painful menstrual flew; urinary incontinence.

PRESENT ILLNESS: This 38-year-old Native American female presented with increased menstrual flow and stress urinary incontinence over the last too years. No other complaints.

PAST MEDICAL HISTORY: Essentially negative except for pyelonefritis as a child with no sequelae. Scarlet fever at age 19 with subsequent tonsilectomy. Has had "sinus trouble" in the past, which cleared after she stopped smoking. (Smoked approximate a pack a day between the ages of 16 and 26 years.)

MEDICATIONS: None. No allergies save for a reaction to ASA.

FAMILY HISTORY: Mother has COPD. Father has hearing lost and elevated cholesterol. One sibling with hearing loss. Maternal aunt with diabetes mellitos, adult onset.

SOCIAL HISTORY: Divorced. Formal smoker (see PMH). Drinks wine socially. Two daughter, aged 6 and 15, in good healthy.

PHYSICAL EXAMINATION: In general, a Well-developed, well-nourished, obese American Indian woman with stable vitals. HEENT: Normocephalic, atraumatic. No neck masses. CHEST: Clear to PNA. HEART: Not enlarge, regular rate and rhythm. No murmurs. BREASTS: No masses. ABDOMEN: Soft, nontender. No organomegaly. PELVIC: Six-centimeter superficial cyst, right upper labia minora. Cystocele.

(Continued)

HISTORY AND PHYSICAL EXAMINATION
Patient Name: Christina Youngblood
Hospital No.: 71210
Page 2

Uterus normal sized with mile prolapse. Cervix oval, clean. Adnexa, cul de sac clean. RECTAL: Confirmatory. EXTREMITIES: Pulses 2+, no edema.

DISPOSITION: Admit for possible bladder repair and hysterectomy.

_____
                        Cynthia Richards, M.D.

CR:xx
D:06/24/- - - -
T:06/25/- - - -

Proofreading Exercise 10

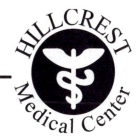

Student _____ (15 errors)

DISCHARGE SUMMARY

Patient Name: Kurt G. Kinsey

Hospital No.: 31498

Admitted: 07/21/- - - -

Discharged: 07/26/- - - -

Consultations: None.

Procedures: Bilateral correcton of hallux valgus with osteotomy, right; Akin procedure, left.

Complications: None.

Admitting Diagnoses: Bilateral hallux valgus.

This 15-year-old young men was admitted for scheduled surgery as listed above.

LABORATORY DATA ON ADMISSION: WBC 6.5, RBC 4.53, hemoglobin 14.1, hematocrit 41, MCV 92, MCH 31.1, MCHC 3.2, platelets 26100; differential, 42 polys, 40 limps, 3 bands, 10 monos, 5 eos. Urinalysis, clear yellow with specific gravity 1.025, PH 5, glucose negative, keytones negative, bilirubin negative. No red cells, no white cells, urobilinogen normal. RPR nonreactive. Postoperative chest film normally.

HOSPITAL COURSE: Patient response to anesthesia uneventfully. Postoperatively patient was hemody-namically stable, afebrile. Physical therapy was instituted during hospital stayed. Therapist taught the patient to use crutches, including on stares and at curbs. Patient did well postoperatively and with the visual thera-py.

DISCHARGE DIAGNOSIS: Bilateral hallux valgus, corrected.

DISCHARGE INSTRUCTIONS: He was discharged on postoperative day five in improved condition to be seen in the office or dressing check in one week. He was given Tylenol No. 3 p.r.n. pain. Diet regular.

(Continued)

DISCHARGE SUMMARY
Patient Name: Kurt G. Kinsey
Hospital No.: 31498
Page 2

Activities: Crutches, no weightbearing, keep lower limbs iced and elevation as much as possible.

_____

Bill Perry, M.D.

BP:xx
D:07/26/- - - -
T:08/02/- - - -

Appendix

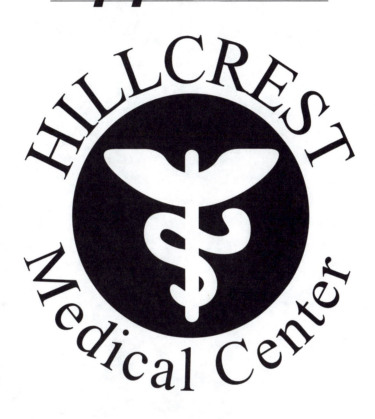

Appendix

PROOFREADER'S MARKS

Defined		Examples

Defined

Paragraph   ¶

Insert a character   ∧

Delete   *e*

Do not change   *stet* or

Transpose   *tr*

Move to the left   [

Move to the right   ]

No paragraph   *no* ¶

Delete and close up   ⌒*e*

Set in caps   *caps* or ≡

Set in lower case   *lc*

Insert a period   ⊙

Quotation marks   ⋁⋁

Comma   ⋀

Insert space   #

Apostrophe   ⋁

Hyphen   =

Close up   ⌒

Use superior figure   ⋁

Set in italic   *ital.* or ___

Move up   ⌐¬

Move down   ⌊⌋

Examples

Begin a new paragraph at this point. Insert a letter here.

Delete these words. Disregard the previous correction. To transpose is to around turn.

Move this copy to the left.

Move this copy to the right.

Do not begin a new paragraph here. Delete the hyphen from pre-empt and close up the space.

a sentence begins with a capital letter. This Word should not be capitalized. Insert a period

Quotation marks and a comma should be placed here he said.

Space between these words. An apostrophe is whats needed here.

Add a hyphen to African American. Close up the extra space.

Footnote this sentence. Set the words, sine qua non, in italics.

This word is too low. That word is too high.

CHALLENGING MEDICAL WORDS, PHRASES, PREFIXES

Each of the following words/abbreviations can be difficult or confusing. Some sound alike yet have different meanings, whereas others do not sound alike but are often used and spelled incorrectly. When listening to dictation, MTs should be aware of regional accent pronunciation as well as foreign accent pronunciation. Be prepared to spell, transcribe, and use *each* of the following terms and abbreviations correctly.

abduction—moving or drawing away

adduction—moving or drawing toward

addiction—habitual dependence that is beyond voluntary control

affect—noun; a state of mind or mood; countenance

affect—verb; to influence, to produce an effect on

effect—noun; result, impression

effect—verb; to result in, bring about, to accomplish

ala nasi—singular noun meaning naris or opening of the nasal cavity

alae nasi—plural noun meaning nares or openings of the nasal cavity

ante—prefix meaning before, in front of, prior, earlier

anti—prefix meaning against, opposite, over

anterior—in front of, forward part of, toward the head

inferior—below, beneath, directed downward, lower surface

interior—inside, inward, inner part or cavity

appose—to place side by side or next to; before, beside, or on

oppose—to place opposite or against something, so as to provide resistance, counterbalance, or contrast

arteritis—inflammation of an <u>artery</u>.

arthritis—inflammation of a joint

aura—subjective evidence of the beginning of either a seizure-like episode or a migraine headache

aural—relating to the ears or to an aura

oral—relating to the mouth

auxiliary—subordinate, secondary

axillary—referring to the underarm area (sometimes temperature is taken there)

bases—plural of basis

basis—the lower, basic, or fundamental part of an object

bile—fluid secreted by the liver

bowel—intestine

Betagan®—an ophthalmologic medication

Betagen®—a surgical scrub

bisect—to cut in half

resect—to cut out a large portion

transect—to cut across

dissect—to cut up, as at autopsy (NOTE: the double "s")

caliber—the diameter of a hollow, tubular structure (like a bullet)

caliper—instrument used for measuring diameters, like pelvic diameters

cancer—cellular tumor, usually malignant

carcinoma—malignant new growth (used in the same way as cancer)

CA—abbreviation for carcinoma or cancer but can also stand for cardiac arrest, coronary artery, and other phrases

Ca—chemical symbol for calcium

callous—adjective meaning hard or bony

callus—noun meaning bone

Carrisyn® (generic is acemannan)—an antiviral, AIDS drug

Carrasyn Hydrogel® (brand name)—a wound dressing, over the counter

chord—a musical word

cord—an anatomic word, e.g., spinal cord

cor—an anatomic word, the heart

cirrhosal—adjective describing a diseased liver

serosal—adjective describing a membrane covering certain cavities of the body

clavicle—collarbone

pedicle—stalk

coarse—rough

course—route, plan

defer—to put off or delay, as in "exam was deferred"

differ—to be unalike or distinct; different

diffuse—adjective meaning scattered, not localized, e.g., diffuse infiltrates

defuse—verb meaning to make a situation less harmful, to calm a crisis

diploic—adjective meaning double

diploë—noun meaning loose bony tissue between the cranial bones

discreet—showing good judgment, prudent (not necessarily a medical word)

discrete—made up of separate parts, not blended; e.g., a discrete mass (NOTE: discrete and separate both end in "te")

disease—morbid process with train of symptoms

sign—evidence of disease that is seen (objective)

symptom—evidence of disease not seen (subjective)

syndrome—a set of symptoms

diverticulum, datum, and medium are each singular nouns taking singular verbs

diverticula, data, and media are each plural nouns—don't forget the plural verb

efflux—outward flow

reflux—backward or return flow

endogenous—growing, developing, or originating from within

exogenous—developing or originating from the outside, e.g., exogenous obesity

enterocleisis—closure of an intestinal wound

enteroclysis—injection of a nutrient or medicinal liquid into the bowel

Erex®—a urologic tablet

Eurax®—a dermatologic cream

Urex®—a urologic tablet

excise—to cut out or off

incise—to cut into

extirpation—to remove entirely, as in extirpation of varicose veins

extubation—to remove a tube, like a nasogastric tube, from a patient

expiration—synonym for death

fecal sac versus thecal sac—theca is an enclosing case or sheath, and both are good phrases

fundus—bottom or base; the part of a hollow organ farthest from its mouth, e.g., the fundus of the stomach

fungus—any one of a class of mushrooms, yeasts, molds

en bloc—in a lump, whole

in situ—in its normal place, confined to the site of origin

in toto—totally

in vivo—within the living body

in vitro—within a test tube (glass)

glans—(singular) a small, rounded mass of gland-like body, e.g., end of penis

glands—(plural) aggregation of cells specialized to secrete or excrete

graft—tissue for implantation (grafting)

graph—a written record, diagram

grasp—grab hold of or seize, as with a surgical instrument

gravida—a pregnant woman (gravida 1 = primigravida)

multiparous—having had two or more pregnancies resulting in viable offspring (para 2 or para 3, etc.)

nulligravida—never having been pregnant

nulliparous—never having given birth to a viable infant

(NOTE: Gravida 5, para 3-1-1-3 refers to a woman who has been pregnant five times, resulting in three full-term deliveries, one premature birth, one abortion or miscarriage, and three living children.

hypo—prefix meaning beneath, under, or deficient

hyper—prefix meaning above, beyond, or excessive

illicit—adjective meaning illegal, as in illicit drugs

elicit—verb meaning to bring out, as to elicit a response or reaction

inflamed, inflammatory, inflammation—same root word; note the spelling difference

ilium—bone (iliac crest)

ileum—portion of the small intestine

ileus—disease (obstruction of small intestine)

NOTE: There is both an iliac artery and an iliac vein.

inter—prefix meaning situated or occurring between

intra—prefix meaning situated or occurring within

infra—prefix meaning situated or occurring beneath

intubated—having had a tube inserted (as into the larynx for providing oxygen)

incubated—placed in an optimal situation for development

lavage—to wash out or irrigate

gavage—forced feeding, especially through a tube

lineal—pertaining to the spleen, as in gastrolineal ligament

renal—pertaining to the kidneys

ligament—a band of tissue connecting bones, supporting viscera

ligature—a thread or wire (suture) for tying vessels

ligate—a verb meaning to sew, tie, or bind with ligature, as after a surgical procedure

liver—the largest gland in the body

livor—the discoloration of the skin on the dependent parts of a corpse

livid—discolored as from a contusion, congestion, or cyanosis

loose—adj. meaning not tight, as in loose clothes

lose—verb meaning to miss from a customary place, as in "Did you lose the book?"

malleus (pl. mallei)—pertaining to the outermost and largest of the three bones in the ear

malleolus (pl. malleoli)—pertaining to the bony prominences on either side of the ankle joint

melena—blood in the stool, remember *melenic stools* is a proper phrase

melanin—dark brown to black pigment

melanotic—pertaining to the presence of melanin or dark pigment in the skin, hair, etc., and has nothing to do with stool

metacarpal—relating to the hand

metatarsal—relating to the foot between the instep and the toes

mucus—noun meaning the free slime of the mucous membrane

mucous—adjective meaning pertaining to or resembling mucus

occur/recur and occurrence/recurrence—something either occurs or recurs; we have an occurrence or a recurrence. (Remember, "reocur" and "reoccurrence" are *not* acceptable, even if dictated. Transcribe recur or recurrence instead.)

ophthalmologist—a physician specializing in the care of the eyes; note spelling, as "ophthal" is often mispronounced and misspelled

os (pl. ora)—the mouth; any opening into a hollow organ or canal; example, cervical os or medication taken per os

os (pl. ossa)—bone; example, os pubis (pubic bone) or ossa cranii (cranial bones)

ostium—(pl. ostia) a small opening

ostiomeatal—*not* osteo, it denotes an opening and has nothing to do with bone

palpation—to touch or feel, examine with the hand(s)

palpitation—rapid and/or irregular pulsations of the heart

para—prefix meaning beside, beyond

peri—prefix meaning around

perineum—genital area, perineal area (between anus and scrotum or vulva)

peritoneum—covering of viscera, lining of abdominopelvic wall

peroneal—pertaining to the fibula, lateral side of the leg, or to the tissues present there

plane—a flat surface

plain—unadorned

pleural—referring to the pleural cavity

plural—meaning more than one

prostate—the male gland surrounding the urethra

prostrate—overcome (prostrate with grief) or lying in a horizontal position

proximal—nearest, closer to any point of reference, a location

approximate—verb meaning to bring close together, as to approximate the edges of a wound

approximately—adverb meaning estimation

pruritus—noun meaning an itchy skin condition

purulent—adjective meaning containing, consisting of, or forming pus—as in a purulent wound

radicle—an anatomic word, the radicles are the smallest branches

radical—going to the root or source of disease, as in radical dissection at surgery

regimen—strictly regulated scheme of diet, exercise, medication, therapy, or training

regime—same as above but pronounced and spelled differently; also used to refer to a government

regiment—a military unit; to organize rigidly

retroperitoneal—adverb meaning behind the peritoneum (a direction)

reperitonealize—verb meaning to cover again with peritoneum

shoddy—inferior goods, hastily or poorly done

shotty—like shot, lead pellets used in shotguns (usually used in reference to lymph nodes, e.g., shotty nodes)

sulfa—pertaining to the sulfonamides, the sulfa drugs

sulfur—brimstone, an element, the symbol for which is S

tendon—noun meaning a band of connective tissue

tendinous—adjective meaning resembling a tendon

tendinitis—noun meaning inflammation of a tendon or tendons (note spelling)

tenia (pl. teniae)—any anatomic bandlike structure

tinea—ringworm, which is a fungus

tinnitus—abnormal noises in the ears, such as ringing or booming or whistling

tonsil, tonsillectomy—same root word; note spelling difference

umbo (pl. umbones)—a round projection, an orthopedic term

umbonate—knoblike

ureter—tube from kidney to bladder; there is a left and a right ureter

urethra—tube carrying urine out of the body; one per person

vagus—noun meaning the tenth cranial nerve or vagus nerve

valgus—adjective meaning bent outward, twisted, deformed

vesicle—little blister or sac

vesical—urinary bladder *only*

villus (pl. villi)—noun meaning little protrusion

villous—adjective meaning shaggy with soft hairs

NOTE: There could be a villous villus.

womb—the uterus

wound—trauma to the body

xerosis—dryness

cirrhosis—liver disease

Proper names for people of different ages include:

neonates or newborns = birth to 1 month of age

infants = 1 month to 2 years of age

children = 2 years to 13 years of age (also boys and girls)

adolescents = 13 years through 17 years of age

adults = 18 years and older (also men and women)

Inflammation is diagnosed when all of the following elements, often referred to as the cardinal signs of inflammation, are present:

calor (heat)

dolor (pain)

rubor (redness)

tumor (swelling)

Reference material used in developing this list includes *Dorland's Illustrated Medical Dictionary,* 28th edition; *Stedman's Medical Dictionary,* 26th edition; *AMA Manual of Style,* 8th edition; *Gregg Reference Manual,* 7th edition, and *The AAMT Book of Style,* c. 1995.

THE LUND BROWDER CHART

The BURN EXTENT ESTIMATOR is a convenient method of estimating the percentage of a patient's burn, the total surface area of the patient's body in square feet, and the approximate surface area of the burn, in square feet.

Shade the burn areas on the figures below, and use the table to estimate the percentage of the burn.

Area	Age—Years					% 2°	% 3°	% Total
	0-1	1-4	5-9	10-15	Adult			
Head	19	17	13	10	7			
Neck	2	2	2	2	2			
Ant. Trunk	13	13	13	13	13			
Post. Trunk	13	13	13	13	13			
R. Buttock	2 1/2	2 1/2	2 1/2	2 1/2	2 1/2			
L. Buttock	2 1/2	2 1/2	2 1/2	2 1/2	2 1/2			
Genitalia	1	1	1	1	1			
R.U. Arm	4	4	4	4	4			
L.U. Arm	4	4	4	4	4			
R.L. Arm	3	3	3	3	3			
L.L. Arm	3	3	3	3	3			
R. Hand	2 1/2	2 1/2	2 1/2	2 1/2	2 1/2			
L. Hand	2 1/2	2 1/2	2 1/2	2 1/2	2 1/2			
R. Thigh	5 1/2	6 1/2	8 1/2	8 1/2	9 1/2			
L. Thigh	5 1/2	6 1/2	8 1/2	8 1/2	9 1/2			
R. Leg	5	5	5 1/2	6	7			
L. Leg	5	5	5 1/2	6	7			
R. Foot	3 1/2	3 1/2	3 1/2	3 1/2	3 1/2			
L. Foot	3 1/2	3 1/2	3 1/2	3 1/2	3 1/2			
				TOTAL				

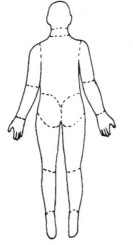

Burn Evaluation
Severity of Burn

1° =

2° =

3° =

REFERENCE MATERIAL

Medical transcriptionists recognize the importance of maintaining a library of reference material. Keeping current is an ongoing and expensive effort; however, having current editions and up-to-date reference material is critical to the accuracy of medical transcription.

Building a Library

Some considerations for building and maintaining a library of reference materials are as follows:

1. Build up a basic library before branching out to the specialty areas, unless you happen to work in one of the specialty or sub-specialty areas.

2. Have available both unabridged and collegiate editions of dictionaries, preferably with copyright dates within the past 5 to 8 years.

3. The word book(s) you choose should illustrate proper word division, i.e., hyphenation at the end of a line for both English and medical words.

4. Medical transcription is a mixture of technical writing and business writing—obtain reference books that will familiarize you with both areas.

5. Write to medical publishing companies and pharmaceutical companies and ask that your name be added to their mailing lists. Your local library will have addresses for companies that publish allied health reference material.

6. Read reviews of newly published editions and ask your peers, coworkers, and professional associates about them before you purchase additional reference books for your library. Some publishing companies offer a trial period on newly purchased volumes.

7. Before you purchase any dictionary or reference work, check for the most recent copyright date. Publishing company personnel can tell you if they plan to have a revision on the market soon; if possible, wait and purchase the new edition.

8. If you enroll in an anatomy, physiology, medical terminology, medical transcrip-

tion, grammar review, or proofreading/editing class, keep your textbooks because they are excellent reference books to add to your library.

9. Medical transcriptionists constantly edit and proofread; therefore, become familiar with the basics in these areas by enrolling in classes and obtaining and reading reference material. Learn the basic proofreading marks; they are printed in grammar reference books, style manuals, in some English dictionaries, and on page XXX in this appendix.

Some publishing companies have developed a series of reference books for MTs in an attempt to meet the needs of the profession. The following list of reference material, which is not all inclusive, contains widely used volumes in several different disciplines.

Abbreviation Books

Common Medical Abbreviations (DeSousa), Delmar Publishers

Medical Abbreviations and Eponyms (Sloane), W.B. Saunders Co.

Medical Abbreviations: 12,000 Conveniences at the Expense of Communications and Safety (Davis), Neil M. Davis Associates

Stedman's Abbreviations, Acronyms & Symbols, Williams & Wilkins

Cardiology/Pulmonary

Cardiology Words and Phrases, Health Professions Institute

Stedman's Cardiology and Pulmonary Words, Williams & Wilkins

Dermatology/Immunology

Stedman's Dermatology & Immunology Words, Williams & Wilkins

HIV Manual for Health Care (Muma) Appleton & Lange

Drug Books

Delmar's A–Z Nurse's Drug Reference (Spratto and Woods) Delmar Publishers

American Drug Index (Billups), Facts and Comparisons

Essentials of Pharmacology for Health Occupations (Woodrow), Delmar Publishers

Physicians' Desk Reference, Physicians Desk Reference, 1998

Physicians' Desk Reference for Nonprescription Drugs, Physicians Desk Reference

Physicians' Desk Reference for Ophthalmology, Physicians Desk Reference

Quick Look Drug Book, Williams & Wilkins

English Dictionaries

Merriam-Webster's Collegiate Dictionary, 10th Edition, Merriam-Webster, Inc.

Webster's Third New International Dictionary, Unabridged, Merriam-Webster, Inc.

Gastroenterology/Genitourinary

GI Words & Phrases, Health Professions Institute

Stedman's GI & GU Words, Williams & Wilkins

General Medicine

Current Medical Terminology (Pyle), Health Professions Institute

H&P: A Nonphysician's Guide to the Medical History and Physical Examination (Dirckx), Health Professions Institute

Medical Word Book, The (Sloane), W.B. Saunders Co.

Stedman's Medical Equipment Words, Williams & Wilkins

Grammar Review/Style Manuals

AAMT Book of Style for Medical Transcription, The (Tessier), AAMT

American Medical Association Manual of Style, Williams & Wilkins

Delmar's Medical Transcription Handbook 2e (Blake), Delmar Publishers 1998

Gregg Reference Manual, The (Sabin), McGraw-Hill

Medical Transcription Guide: Do's and Don'ts (Fordney/Diehl), W.B. Saunders Co.

Laboratory/Pathology

Laboratory Medicine: Essentials of Anatomic and Clinical Pathology (Dirckx), Health Professions Institute

Stedman's Pathology & Lab Medicine Words, Williams & Wilkins

Word Book in Pathology & Laboratory Medicine, A (Sloane/Dusseau), W.B. Saunders Co.

Understanding Laboratory and Diagnostic Tests (Moisio & Moisio) Delmar Publishers, 1998

Medical Dictionaries

Dorland's Illustrated Medical Dictionary, W.B. Saunders Co.

Stedman's Medical Dictionary, Williams & Wilkins

Medical Terminology/Anatomy and Physiology

Medical Terminology for Health Professions, 3e (Ehrlich), Delmar Publishers, 1997

Medical Terminology: A Programmed Text, 7e (Smith, Davis, Denner II), Delmar Publishers, 1995

Essentials of Medical Terminology (Davies) Delmar Publishers, 1998

Medical Terminology CD-ROM: A Visual Guide (Masters), Delmar Publishers, 1997

Body Structures and Functions (Fong/Scott), Delmar Publishers

Color Atlas of Human Anatomy (McMinn/Hutchings), Mosby-Year Book, Inc.

Terminology for Allied Health Professionals (Sormunen/Moisio), Delmar Publishers

Understanding Human Anatomy and Physiology (Solomon/Phillips), W.B. Saunders Co.

Obstetrics/Gynecology

Stedman's OB/GYN Words, Williams & Wilkins

Oncology

Stedman's Radiology & Oncology Words, Williams & Wilkins

Ophthalmology

Dictionary of Eye Terminology (Cassin/Solomon), Triad Publishing Co.

Orthopedics/Neurology/Rehabilitation

Orthopedic/Neurology Words & Phrases, Health Professions Institute

Stedman's Orthopaedic & Rehab Words, Williams & Wilkins

Periodicals

JAAMT (Journal of the American Association for Medical Transcription), AAMT (bimonthly)

Medical Transcription Student Network Gazette, Health Professions Institute (quarterly)

Perspectives on the Medical Transcription Profession, Health Professions Institute (quarterly)

Psychiatry

Psychiatric Words & Phrases (D'Onofrio), Health Professions Institute

Psychiatry Word Book with Street Talk Terms, The (Forbis), F.A. Davis

Radiology

Stedman's Radiology/Oncology Words, Williams & Wilkins

Radiology Words & Phrases, Health Professions Institute

Word Book in Radiology (Sloane), W.B. Saunders Co.

Surgery

Stedman's Medical Equipment Words, Williams & Wilkins

Surgical Word Book, The (Tessier), W.B. Saunders Co.

Syllabus for the Surgeon's Secretary (Szulec), Medical Arts Publishing

Publishers

AAMT (American Association for Medical Transcription), PO Box 576187, Modesto, CA 95357-6187; phone 209-551-0883 or 800-982-2182; FAX 209-551-9317

Appleton & Lange, PO Box 120041, Stamford, CT 06912-0041; phone 800-423-1359; FAX 203-406-4600

Delmar Publishers, PO Box 15015, Albany, NY 12212-5015; phone 800-347-7707; FAX 518-464-0301

Facts and Comparisons, 111 West Port Plaza, Suite 400, St. Louis, MO 63141; phone 800-223-0554; FAX 314-878-5563

Health Professions Institute, PO Box 801, Modesto, CA 95353; phone 209-551-2112; FAX 209-551-0404

McGraw-Hill, Blue Ridge Summit, PA 17294; phone 800-262-4729; FAX 614-759-3644

Medical Arts Publishing Co., PO Box 36600, Grosse Pointe, MI 48236

Merriam-Webster, Inc., 47 Federal Street, Springfield, MA 01102; phone 800-828-1880; FAX 413-731-5979

Mosby-Year Book, Inc., 11830 Westline Industrial Drive, St. Louis, MO 63146; phone 800-426-4545; FAX 800-535-9935

Neil M. Davis Associates, 1143 Wright Drive, Huntingdon Valley, PA 19006; phone 215-947-1752; FAX 215-938-1937

Physicians Desk Reference, PO Box 10689, Des Moines, IA 50336; phone 800-232-7379; FAX 201-573-4956

Triad Publishing Co., PO Drawer 13355, Gainesville, FL 32604-1355; phone 904-373-5800; FAX 904-373-1488

W. B. Saunders Co., 6277 Sea Harbor Drive, Orlando, FL 32887; phone 800-545-2522, 800-433-0001 (FL); FAX 800-874-6418

Williams & Wilkins, Waverly, Inc., 351 W. Camden Street, Baltimore, MD 21201-2436; phone 800-527-5597; FAX 800-447-8438

Transcription Web Sites

Web sites come and go and addresses change frequently. Here are a few to investigate:

http://www.mtdesk.com—This site has links to manufacturers, sample reports, and a bulletin board where you can leave a message if you have a word you can't find.

http://www.rxlist.com—Comprehensive listing of medications. You can even look with a phonetic spelling or key in a diagnosis to help you find the drug.

http://www.helix.com—You have to register to use this site, but it's free. It's a good general medical research site.

http://www.medmatrix.org/index.asp—Another free site, but you have to register to use it. You can research medical literature through this site.

http://www.mtmonthly.com—This site lists terms, drugs, instruments, and some specialty lists, like AIDS terms and herbs used in alternative medicine.

A HEALTHCARE CONTROLLED VOCABULARY

From *Medical Abbreviations: 12,000 Conveniences at the Expense of Communications and Safety*, Eighth Edition, by Neil M. Davis (Huntingdon Valley, PA: Neil M. Davis Associates, 1997) Reprinted with permission.

Presently there are no standards for physician's orders, consultations, written prescriptions, standing orders, computer order sets, nurse's medication administration records, pharmacy profiles, hospital formularies, etc. Because in the healthcare field everyone does their own thing, there are many variations. These variations in the way abbreviations are expressed are not always understood and at times are misinterpreted. They cause delays in initiating therapy, cause accidents, waste time for everyone in clarifying these documents, lengthen the time it takes to train those working in the healthcare field, lengthen hospital stays, and waste money.

A controlled vocabulary similar to what is used in the aviation industry is needed. Everyone in the aviation industry "follows the book," and uses a controlled vocabulary. All pilots and air traffic controllers say, "alpha", "bravo", "charley." They do not go off on their own and say "adam", "beef", "candy!" They say "one three," not thirteen, because thirteen sounds like thirty. Radio transmission in the aviation industry is not easy to decipher, yet because precision is critical everything possible is done to eliminate error. To prevent errors all radio transmissions are given only in English, every transmission is given in the same order, and must be immediately repeated by the receiver to make sure it was heard correctly. Written and oral communication in the medical professions are just

as critical and are also not easy to decipher, so establishing a controlled vocabulary is also necessary in this industry.

Listed below are three organizations that have ongoing projects related to standardizing medical terminology:

Computer-Based Patient Record Institute, Inc.
1000 East Woodfield Rd. Suite 102
Schaumburg, IL 60173

The United States Pharmacopeial Convention, Inc.
12601 Twinbrook Parkway
Rockville, MD 20852

National Library of Medicine
Unified Medical Language System
8600 Rockville Pike
Bethesda, MD 20894

Listed below is the start of a Healthcare Controlled Vocabulary. The basis for this controlled vocabulary is established standard terminology and the result of 30 years of studying medication errors by this author.

It is anticipated that a Healthcare Controlled Vocabulary, with professional organizations' input and backing, will grow and some day evolve into an "official standard." Your suggestions and comments are vital to this growth and eventual recognition. It is always safest to avoid the use of abbreviations unless a standard has been established and is well publicized in your work environment.

Standard	What not to use or do	Comments
100 mg (100 space mg)	100mg (100 no space mg)	A USP* standard way of expressing a strength is to leave a space between the number and its units. Leaving this space makes it easier to read the number as can be seen below. 1mg 1 mg 10mg 10 mg 100mg 100 mg
1 mg	1.0 mg	This is a USP standard. When a trailing zero is used, the decimal point is sometimes not seen thus causing a tenfold overdose. These overdoses have caused injury and death.
0.1 mL	.1 mL	When the decimal point is not seen, this is read as 1 mL, causing a tenfold overdose.
once daily (Do not abbreviate.)	The abbreviation OD The abbreviation QD	The classic meaning for OD is right eye. Liquids intended to be given once daily are mistakenly given in the right eye. When the Q is dotted too aggressively it looks like Q.I.D. and the medication is given four times daily. When a lower case q is used, the tail of the q has come up between the q and the d to make it look like qid. In the United Kingdom, Q.D. means four times daily
unit (Do not abbreviate. Write "unit" using a lower-case u)	The abbreviation U	The handwritten U is mistaken for a zero when poorly written causing a tenfold overdose (i.e., 6 U regular insulin is read as 60). The poorly written U has also been read as a 4, 6 and cc. Write "unit," leaving a space between the number and the word unit.
mg (Lower case mg with no period)	mg., Mg., Mg, MG, mgm, mgs	The USP standard expression is the mg
mL (lower case m with a capital L, no period)	mL., ml, ml., mls, mLs, cc	The USP standard expression is the mL
Use generic names or trademarks	Do not abbreviate drug names or combinations of drugs, such as CPZ, PBZ, NTG, MS, 5FC, MTX, 6MP, MOPP, ASA, HCTZ, etc. Do not use shortened names or chemical names	Abbreviated drug names and acronyms are not always known to the reader, at times they have more than one possible meaning, or are thought to be another drug. When the chemical name "6 mercaptopurine" has been used, six doses of mercaptopurine have been mistakenly administered. The generic name, mercaptopurine, should be used. When an unofficial shortened version of the name norfloxacin, norflox was used, Norflex was mistakenly given. An order for Aredia was read as Adriamycin, as some professionals abbreviated the name Adriamycin as "Adria" which looks like Aredia.

Standard	What not to use or do	Comments
The metric system	The apothecary system (grains, drams, minims, ounces, etc.)	The Apothecary system is so rarely used it is not recognized or understood. The symbol for minim (η) is read as mL; the symbol for one dram (℥т) is read as 3 tablespoons, and gr (grain) is read as gram.
Use properly placed commas for numbers above 999, as in 10,000, or 5,000,000	5000000	Many people have difficulty in reading large numbers such as 5000000. The use of commas helps the reader to read these numbers correctly.
600 mg When possible, do not use decimal expressions.	0.6 g	A USP standard. The elimination of decimals lessens the chance for error.
25 mcg	0.025 mg	Mistakes are made when reading numbers less than 1 with decimals.
Do not use the term "bolus" in conjunction with the administration of potassium chloride injection. Use specific concentrations and the time in which the drug should be administered.		Some physicians will erroneously indicate that potassium chloride injection should be "bolused" or be given "IV push," vaguely meaning that it should not be dripped in slowly. Many deaths have been reported when prescribers have been taken literally and the potassium chloride was given by bolus or IV push. Orders should be specific such as, "20 mEq of potassium chloride in 50 mL of 5% dextrose to run over 30 minutes."
use "and"	Do not use a slash mark or the symbol "&"	A slash mark looks like a one. An order written "6 units regular insulin/20 units NPH insulin," was read as 120 units of NPH insulin. The symbol "&" has been read as a 4.
Orally transmitted medical orders should be read back as heard for verification	Do not assume that one has spoken or heard correctly.	During oral communications, speakers misspeak and/or transcribers mishear. To minimize these errors, the transmitter must speak clearly and slowly, the transcriber must repeat what was transcribed, and the transmitter must listen attentively when this is being done. This is less likely to occur when the prescription is complete.
When prescriptions are written or orally transmitted they must be complete. • dosage form must be specified • strength must be specified • directions must be specified • included in the directions must be the purpose or indication.	Incomplete orders	Prescribers on occasion think of one drug and mistakenly order another. Nurses and pharmacists on occasion misread prescriptions because of error, poor handwriting or poor oral communications, or look alike or sound alike drugs.[1] When the prescription is complete and the purpose or indication is included, these errors are less likely to occur. Listing the purpose or indication on the prescription label will assist in increasing patient compliance.

Standard	What not to use or do	Comments
Written communications must be legible.	Illegible handwriting	Prescribers who cannot or will not write legibly must either print (if this would be legible), type, use a computer, or have an employee write for them and then immediately verify and sign the document.
Prescribe specific doses.	Do not prescribe 2 ampuls or 2 vials	There are often more than one size or concentration of drug available. Failing to be specific will lead to unintended doses being administered.
Establish a list of approved abbreviations with no abbreviation having more than one possible meaning within a context.	Everyone using their own abbreviations	To understand the scope of this problem examine the contents of this book for abbreviations that have many meanings and for obscure abbreviations that would not generally be recognized.
Use h or hr for hour	°	An order written as q 4° has been read as q 40 or the symbol ° has not been understood.

*USP = United States Pharmacopeia

1. Da vis NM, Cohen MR, Teplitsky BS. Look-alike and sound alike drug names: The problem and the solution. Hosp Pharm 1992:27:95-110

Index

HOW TO USE THE COMPUTER SOFTWARE DISK

The 3.5" computer software disk is included to help you study and practice medical transcription. The disk contains standard report templates for use in transcription exercises, eight on-line Matching Exercises designed to enhance your familiarity with medical terminology, ten Wordfind Puzzles, and six Proofreading exercises. The report templates have been prepared for use in multiple versions of Corel® WordPerfect® (versions 6.1 through 8), and Microsoft® Word (versions 6.0 through 97).

System Requirements

386 Processor or better
Windows® 3.1, Windows 95 or newer, Windows NT™
4 MB RAM
2 MB free hard disk space
3.5" disk drive
Mouse

Installing the Hillcrest Software

1. Insert the Hillcrest Medical Center disk into your computer's 3.5" disk drive (usually this is disk drive A: or B:).

2. Choose **Start** in Windows taskbar at the bottom left corner of your computer screen, and then choose **Run...**

   -or-

   If you are using Windows 3.1, in the **Windows Program Manager** choose **File** and then choose **Run**.

3. In the Run window, type **A:\SETUP** (or B:\SETUP if your disk is in drive B:), and click **OK**.

4 Read the setup Welcome screen, and choose click **Next** to proceed. Then click **Next** again to accept the default location for the Hillcrest program to be installed on your computer hard disk.

5. When installation is complete, you will see an information screen telling you so. Click OK.

You are now ready to run the program. Don't forget to remove the program installation disk from the disk drive.

Getting Started

After the program has been installed you can launch it by choosing **Start > Programs > Delmar Applications > Hillcrest Med. Center**
-or-
If you are using Windows 3.1, double click the Hillcrest Med. Center icon in the Program Manager window.

We recommend that as you work, you have a "work" disk available on which to save your transcription reports.

When you first load the program, explore Help on the top menu bar to learn how to navigate through the program and take advantage of its features and reports. In addition to finding user instructions in Help, you will also find a list of physicians/practitioners referred to in the transcription exercizes. The list is provided as reference so that you will know how to spell their names when you are transcribing a report.

See also the Preface of this book for Report Formatting Guidelines and tips for using Corel® WordPerfect® and Microsoft® Word keyboard commands.

Removing the Program from your Hard Disk

If you ever wish to remove the Hillcrest program from your hard disk, you may do so by choosing Start > Programs > Delmar Applications > UnInstall Hillcrest.

Trademarks

Microsoft and Windows are registered trademarks of Microsoft Corporation. Corel and WordPerfect are registered trademarks of Corel Corporation.

License Agreement for Delmar Publishers
an International Thomson Publishing company

Educational Software/Data

You the customer, and Delmar incur certain benefits, rights, and obligations to each other when you open this package and use the software/data it contains. BE SURE YOU READ THE LICENSE AGREEMENT CAREFULLY, SINCE BY USING THE SOFTWARE/DATA YOU INDICATE YOU HAVE READ, UNDERSTOOD, AND ACCEPTED THE TERMS OF THIS AGREEMENT.

Your rights:

1. You enjoy a non-exclusive license to use the enclosed software/data on a single microcomputer that is not operating as a network server or multi-machine system in consideration for payment of the required license fee, (which may be included in the purchase price of an accompanying print component), or receipt of this software/data, and your acceptance of the terms and conditions of this agreement.

2. You own the media on which the software/data is recorded, but you acknowledge that you do not own the software and data recorded on them. You also acknowledge that the software/data is furnished "as is," and contains copyrighted and/or proprietary and confidential information of Delmar Publishers or its licensors.

3. If you do not accept the terms of this license agreement you may return the media within 30 days. However, you may not use the software during this period.

There are limitations on your rights:

1. You may not copy or print the software/data for any reason whatsoever, except to install it on a hard drive on a single microcomputer and to make one archival copy, unless copying or printing is expressly permitted in writing or statements recorded on the diskette(s).

2. You may not revise, translate, convert, disassemble or otherwise reverse engineer the software/data except that you may add to or rearrange any data recorded on the media as part of the normal use of the software/data.

3. You may not sell, license, lease, rent, loan, or otherwise distribute or network the software/data except that you may give the software/data to a student or and instructor for use at school or, temporarily at home.

Should you fail to abide by the Copyright Law of the United States as it applies to this software/data your license to use it will become invalid. You agree to erase or otherwise destroy the software/data immediately after receiving note of Delmar Publishers' termination of this agreement for violation of its provisions.

Delmar Publishers gives you a LIMITED WARRANTY covering the enclosed software/data. The LIMITED WARRANTY can be found in this product and/or the instructor's manual that accompanies it.

This license is the entire agreement between you and Delmar Publishers interpreted and enforced under New York law.

Limited Warranty

Delmar Publishers warrants to the original licensee/purchaser of this copy of microcomputer software/data and the media on which it is recorded that the media will be free from defects in material and workmanship for ninety (90) days from the date of original purchase. All implied warranties are limited in duration to this ninety (90) day period. THEREAFTER, ANY IMPLIED WARRANTIES, INCLUDING IMPLIED WARRANTIES OF MERCHANTABILITY AND FITNESS FOR A PARTICULAR PURPOSE ARE EXCLUDED. THIS WARRANTY IS IN LIEU OF ALL OTHER WARRANTIES, WHETHER ORAL OR WRITTEN, EXPRESSED OR IMPLIED.

If you believe the media is defective, please return it during the ninety day period to the address shown below. A defective diskette will be replaced without charge provided that it has not been subjected to misuse or damage.

This warranty does not extend to the software or information recorded on the media. The software and information are provided "AS IS." Any statements made about the utility of the software or information are not to be considered as express or implied warranties. Delmar will not be liable for incidental or consequential damages of any kind incurred by you, the consumer, or any other user.

Some states do not allow the exclusion or limitation of incidental or consequential damages, or limitations on the duration of implied warranties, so the above limitation or exclusion may not apply to you. This warranty gives you specific legal rights, and you may also have other rights which vary from state to state. Address all correspondence to:

Delmar Publishers
3 Columbia Circle
P. O. Box 15015
Albany, NY 12212-5015